T0332536

PAIN MANAGEMENT OF AIDS PATIENTS

CURRENT MANAGEMENT OF PAIN

P. Prithvi Raj. Series Editor

The series, *Current Management of Pain,* is intended by the series editor and the publishers to provide up-to-date information on advances in the clinical management of acute and chronic pain and related research as quickly as possible. Both the series editor and the publishers felt that, although comprehensive texts are now available, they do not always cover the rapid advances in this field. Another format was needed to publish advances in basic sciences and clinical modalities and to bring them rapidly to the practitioners in the community. A questionnaire was sent to selected clinicians and, based on their responses, topics were chosen by the series editor. Editors of each volume were chosen for their expertise in the field and their ability to encourage other active pain specialists to contribute their knowledge:

Ghia, J.N., ed.: The Multidisciplinary Pain Center: Organization and Personnel Functions for Pain Management, 1988. ISBN 0-89838-359-5.

Lynch, N.T., Vasudevan, S.V.: Persistent Pain: Psychosocial Assessment and Intervention, 1988. ISBN 0-89838-363-3.

Abram, S.E., ed.: Cancer Pain, 1988. ISBN 0-89838-389-7.

Racz, G.B., ed.: Techniques of Neurolysis, 1989. ISBN 0-89838-397-8.

Stanton-Hicks, M., ed.: Pain and the Sympathetic Nervous System, 1989. ISBN 0-7923-0304-0.

Rawal, N., Coombs, D.W., eds.: Spinal Narcotics, 1989. ISBN 0-7923-0374-1.

Stanton-Hicks, M., Janig, W., eds., Reflex Sympathetic Dystrophy, 1989. ISBN 0-7923-0527-2.

Janisse, T., ed.: Pain Management of Aids Patients, 1991. 0-7923-1056-X.

PAIN MANAGEMENT OF AIDS PATIENTS

EDITED BY THOMAS JANISSE

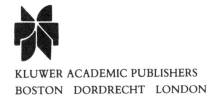

KLUWER ACADEMIC PUBLISHERS
BOSTON   DORDRECHT   LONDON

Distributors for North America:
Kluwer Academic Publishers
101 Philip Drive
Assinippi Park
Norwell, Massachusetts 02061 USA
Distributors for all other countries:
Kluwer Academic Publishers Group
Distribution Centre
Post Office Box 322
3300 AH Dordrecht, THE NETHERLANDS

Library of Congress Cataloging-in-Publication Data

Pain management of AIDS patients / edited by Thomas Janisse.
    p.   cm.—(Current management of pain; 8)
    Includes index.
    ISBN 0-7923-1056-X
    1. AIDS (Disease)—Complications and sequelae—Treatment.
2. Pain—Treatment. 3. Anesthesia. 4. Analgesia. I. Janisse,
Thomas. II. Series.
    [DNLM: 1. Acquired Immunodeficiency Syndrome—therapy.
2. Anesthesia. 3. Pain—prevention & control. W1 CU788LW v. 8 /
WD 308 P144]
RC607.A26P35   1991
616.97'9206—dc20
DNLM/DLC
for Library of Congress   90-15622
                                                                    CIP

Printed on acid-free Paper
Printed in the United States of America.

To my family,
Cherryl, Laura, and Jill,
Emile, Rita, Richard, Joanne, and John.

To P. Prithvi Raj, Jim, Vickie, and Steve.
Who offered me an opportunity.

CONTENTS

Contributing authors   ix

Series editor's comment   xi

Preface   xiii

1. Etiology, pathogenesis, and diagnosis   1
   thomas janisse

2. Psychoneuroimmunology and AIDS   15
   sanford i. cohen,
   susan blumenthaul

3. Anesthetic management of AIDS patients   37
   ernest r. greene, jr.
   thomas janisse

4. Management of the parturient with AIDS   61
   m. joanne douglas

5. Orofacial pain in AIDS patients   73
   douglas w. anderson
   marshall d. bedder

6. Chronic pain syndromes in AIDS patients   91
   richard l. rauck

Index   115

CONTRIBUTING AUTHORS

Douglas W. Anderson
Adjunct Instructor of Anesthesiology
Pain Management Service
Department of Anesthesiology
Oregon Health Sciences University
3181 SW Sam Jackson Park Road
Portland, Oregon 97201

Marshall D. Bedder
Assistant Professor of Anesthesiology
Assistant Professor of Surgery
Division of Neurosurgery
Director, Pain Management Service
Oregon Health Sciences University
3181 SE Sam Jackson Park Road
Portland, Oregon 97201

Susan Blumenthaul
Chief, Behavioral Medicine Program
Health and Behavior Research Branch
Division of Basic Sciences
National Institute of Mental Health
5600 Fishers Lane
Rockville, MD 20857

Sanford I. Cohen
Professor of Psychiatry
Director, Stress and Behavioral
  Medicine Center
Department of Psychiatry
Department of Miami School of
  Medicine
Miami, Florida 33136

M. Joanne Douglas
  Associate Clinical Professor of
  Anaesthesiology
Division of Obstetric Anaesthesia
The University of British Columbia and
  Grace Hospital
4490 Oak Street
Vancouver, British Columbia, Canada
  V6H 3V5

Ernest R. Greene, Jr.
Associate Professor of Anesthesiology
University of Alabama at Birmingham
Chief of Anesthesia

Veterans Administration Medical
Center and Cooper Green Hospital
700 South 19th Street
Birmingham, Alabama 35233

Thomas Janisse
Chief of Anesthesia
Director, Pain Service
Department of Anesthesia
Kaiser Sunnyside Medical Center
10200 SE Sunnyside Road
Clackamas, Oregon 97215

Richard L. Rauck
Assistant Professor of Anesthesiology
Director, Pain Control Center
Bowman Gray School of Medicine
2240 Cloverdale Avenue
Winston Salem, North Carolina 27103

ILLUSTRATOR

Stephen Bachhuber
Staff Anesthesiologist
Department of Anesthesia
Kaiser Sunnyside Medical Center
10200 SE Sunnyside Road
Clackamas, Oregon 97215

Acquired immunodeficiency syndrome has become a significant health problem in the practice of medicine today. While the research in AIDS is being funded and progressing at a rapid rate, the cure for this syndrome is not yet in sight. Most of the advances are in diagnosis and screening of patients with latent AIDS. In addition, literature is profusely replete with its epidemiological consequences and health care cost to the society. As far as this editor knows, no publication is available on the pain syndromes associated with AIDS. Furthermore, the incidence, severity, and duration of such pain syndromes are unknown. It is therefore necessary that pain syndromes caused by AIDS should be addressed and evaluated and the therapeutic plans rationalized for this unfortunate group of patients.

Tom Janisse has undertaken this task and with the help of his coauthors, produced an excellent monograph that is unique and, I hope, useful for decreasing the suffering of AIDS patients.

Prithvi Raj

Thousands of articles and many books have been published on the acquired immunodeficiency syndrome (AIDS). There are, however, no studies or case reports and only several articles published on the anesthetic considerations for a person with AIDS or in pain with AIDS. There is no literature on the pain management of AIDS patients. Writing on this subject must be considered trailblazing.

The reason anesthesiologists should know about AIDS has rapidly extended from concern over transmission of infection to anesthetic and analgesic considerations. The anesthesiologist may also be part of a pain management team on either an acute or a chronic pain service. The requirement may be to treat an HIV-positive or AIDS patient acutely postoperatively or in consult to a psychiatric, medical, or surgical service. In a pain clinic setting, the anesthesiologist may be concerned with diagnosis, treatment, or referral for other multidisciplinary consultation.

The earlier question of central nervous system involvement in AIDS is now moot, rapidly replaced with the knowledge that the CNS, if not primarily infected, is so shortly thereafter. Protected by the blood-brain barrier, the CNS becomes both a sanctuary and reservoir for HIV. Because neurologic complications of HIV are common, and since knowledge of the nervous system is essential for anesthetic and pain management, it is important to review HIV infection of the nervous system. In chapter 1, I introduce the subject of HIV infection and discuss the significant nervous system alterations as a foundation for the discussions in the following chapters.

Acquired immunodeficiency syndrome is both a viral immune disorder and a neuropsychiatric disorder. Its development and course appears to be a multifactorial process, with many "co-factors" either defined or proposed. This state fits the "biopsychosocial" model of disease that considers the interaction of genetic, biological, emotional, behavioral, situational, and cultural factors in the pathogenesis of all disease. The traditional biomedical "mind-body" model, which ignores the many other potential components of health and disease and their impact, cannot alone serve the AIDS dilemma. Because of recent proposals that psychosocial factors may exacerbate HIV infection, it becomes increasingly important for us to know of these interactions and to refer those people infected with HIV for evaluation and treatment by mental health providers. Largely because of the AIDS crisis, the biopsychosocial model of disease has become more widely recognized as essential in the management of people with any illness. In chapter 2, Drs. Cohen and Blumenthaul review the research that forms the foundation for this field and the recent clinical studies of those people with HIV infection.

Development of an anesthetic plan and delivery of the anesthetic require special consideration of the technical aspects and the drug management of persons infected with HIV. Further, only recently have anesthesiologists routinely elected to deliver an intraoperative regional anesthetic instead of a general anesthetic and to offer those people regional postoperative analgesia managed by an acute pain service. The person with HIV infection would benefit from a carefully administered conventional anesthetic, as well as from these new services, but presents the anesthesiologist or pain specialist with new pathophysiologic variables. In chapter 3, Dr. Greene and I discuss general and regional anesthetic management for the person with HIV infection.

A pregnant woman with HIV infection presents numerous questions and potential problems. What are the effects of HIV infection on women? How does HIV infection alter the course of pregnancy? How does pregnancy alter the course of HIV infection? What are the effects of HIV infection on the fetus and on the mother? These and other specific issues regarding the parturient with HIV infection Dr. Douglas addresses in chapter 4. Most interesting are the results of a survey conducted by Dr. Douglas at the annual meeting of the Society for Obstetric Anesthesia and Perinatology on the current anesthetic management of the pain of labor and delivery in those parturients with HIV infection.

The anesthesiologist, pain management specialist, and the dentist all benefit from knowing about orofacial disorders secondary to HIV infection, because several are common, they can be the initial presentation of HIV infection, and transmission may occur with oral or airway manipulation. In chapter 5, Drs. Anderson and Bedder offer a comprehensive presentation on this subject.

Many people with HIV infection and AIDS are beginning to live longer, and studies are following "long survivors." An increasing number of people require management of pain that has become chronic. In chapter 6, Dr. Rauck examines the diagnosis and treatment of chronic pain syndromes secondary to HIV infection. This chapter offers pain management techniques that may complement traditional medical treatment or that may have new application in people with HIV infection or AIDS.

The authors of this book take the first look at pain management of AIDS patients and those with early HIV infection. Their investigation, clinical experience, and insight provide exceptional material for study and improved practice of pain management. Of greatest importance is the potential benefit to people who experience pain either perioperatively or secondary to disease process. We hope this book helps them.

PAIN MANAGEMENT OF AIDS PATIENTS

1. ETIOLOGY, PATHOGENESIS, AND DIAGNOSIS

THOMAS JANISSE

Acquired immunodeficiency syndrome (AIDS) is caused by a virus now called the human immunodeficiency virus type 1 (HIV-1).[1, 2] In 1986 a second virus, HIV-2, was discovered that causes an immunodeficiency state clinically indistinguishable from that caused by HIV-1.[3] This finding is important since HIV-2 may not be detected by routine screening tests for HIV-1. Terminology has changed to parallel medical advances so that it is now more accurate to consider a wide spectrum of HIV infection, from apparently healthy asymptomatic people to those in the advanced state of AIDS.

Human immunodeficiency virus type 1 is a retrovirus containing RNA, core proteins, and a reverse transcriptase enzyme, which allow the virus to assemble DNA from its RNA. The new viral DNA incorporates into the host DNA, encoding for viral replication. The RNA contains genes that regulate HIV synthesis, determine virus infectivity, and down-regulate HIV replication.[4]

The surface glycoprotein of HIV binds with an antigenic receptor molecule, called CD4+, on the surface of other cells: the lymphocyte, the monocyte-macrophage, and central nervous system (CNS) cells. When infected the helper-inducer T lymphocytes (T4) become dysfunctional and die, resulting in an increasing lymphopenia and in secondary dysfunction in the other lymphocytes that it interacts with (the suppressor T cell and the B cell). Generalized lymphocyte dysfunction results in immune system defects and incompetence.[5] The monocyte-macrophage cells are not readily killed by the

HIV and so may act as a reservoir for HIV and a transport vehicle to the CNS.[6]

The HIV infection may be latent, slowly progressive, or rapidly progressive. The rate of change appears to be secondary to activation by antigenic stimulation from various potential sources, including coinfections, genetic predisposition, environmental factors, and other unknown mechanisms.[7]

Cell-mediated immunity is profoundly affected by HIV infection, permitting the development of opportunistic infection secondary to both a deficiency in T-cell number and function. Commonly, the ratio of helper-inducer to suppressor T cells (T4/T8 ratio) decreases. Although B-cell function may be abnormal, elevated serum immunoglobulins are a common finding.[8] This immunodeficiency disorder presents clinically in several different forms, as shown in table 1–1, which is a modified list of Saxon and Campen.[9]

Currently, HIV infection is diagnosed by serologic testing or, if a person is symptomatic, by meeting the Centers for Disease Control's 1987 revision of surveillance case definition for AIDS.[10] The HIV antibody test, both remarkably specific and sensitive, is an enzyme-linked immunosorbent assay (ELISA). If positive on repeat ELISA testing, a more specific confirmatory test, the Western blot, is performed.[11]

NERVOUS SYSTEM

Pathogenesis

The earlier question of CNS involvement in AIDS is now moot, having been rapidly replaced with the knowledge that the CNS, if not primarily infected, is so shortly thereafter. Protected by the blood-brain barrier, the CNS becomes both a sanctuary and reservoir for HIV. Neurologic complications of HIV were initially reported in 1983 as 30%,[12] then in 1987 as 63%, in patients with AIDS or AIDS-related complex (ARC).[13] Autopsy-based studies in the same year found 80% of adult AIDS patients with neuropathological abnormalities[14] and 90% of AIDS or ARC patients with subacute encephalitis.[15]

Table 1–1. General patterns of presentations of HIV infection

---

 1. Aysmptomatic
 2. Acute HIV disease (acute viral infection)
 3. Lymphadenopathy
 4. Severe opportunistic infections (pneumocystis)
 5. Mild opportunistic infections (mucocutaneous Candida)
 6. Opportunistic tumors (Kaposi's sarcoma)
 7. Autoimmune disorders (idiopathic thrombocytopenia purpura)
 8. Systemic symptoms only (fever, chills, and fatigue)
 9. Neurologic disease (HIV encephalopathy)
10. Psychiatric disorders (major depression)
11. Renal disease (HIV nephropathy)

Source: Saxon and Campen.[9]

Table 1–2. Postulated etiopathogenesis of HIV encephalopathy

1. Neuronal death resulting directly from HIV infection
2. Neuronal dysfunction, without cell death, resulting from neuronal HIV infection
3. Alteration of CNS trophic factors, such as nerve growth factor, resulting in neuronal death or dysfunction
4. Alteration of CNS neurotransmitter production or release
5. Virus blocks neurotransmitter or trophic factor receptor sites, resulting in cellular dysfunction or death
6. Elaboration of intrathecal humoral immunomodulators, such as alpha interferon and interleukin 2A, that result in altered neuronal function or survival

Source: Berger.[16]

Neurologic disease can be either a direct result of HIV or a direct or indirect result of HIV immunosuppression. The former will be expanded upon next. The latter includes opportunistic infections, neoplasms, metabolic-nutritional disorders, and vascular complications (which will be considered under Regional Anesthetic Management in chapter 3).

The etiology of the nervous system pathogenesis of HIV infection remains a dilemma for those who would treat it. Basic to the problem is the discrepancy between the extent of HIV CNS pathology and the resultant clinical disease. There can be either significant pathology and little clinical impairment or insignificant pathology and great clinical impairment. An example of the latter is clinically dramatic HIV encephalopathy with minimal neuronal death. The primary cause appears to be neuron or neurotransmitter dysfunction. Berger listed the postulated mechanisms[16], as shown in table 1–2.

Neurotransmitter dysfunction relates specifically to studies of a shared intercellular network joining the brain, glands, and immune system. One such study proposes that AIDS and its dementia are a neuropeptide disorder.[17] Psychoneuroimmunology has produced clinical studies supporting this interaction, which will be discussed in detail in chapter 2.

Trophism

Initially, HIV was considered primarily "lymphotrophic," since it preferentially replicated in the CD4+ helper T lymphocyte.[18] Now, based on HIV affinity for brain macrophages,[19] and HIV strains distinctly associated with neurological disease apart from immune deficiency,[20] HIV is recognized as equally "neurotrophic." Significant support for this is provided by the numerous neurological presentations of HIV and the extent of neurologic disease among HIV-positive individuals.

CENTRAL NERVOUS SYSTEM

Clinical manifestations and syndromes

At the time of acute HIV infection, there may be a transient HIV antigenemia, with HIV antibody seroconversion following in eight to twelve weeks but possibly not occurring for several months.[21] Acute clinical manifestations may appear after a three- to six-week incubation period and include fever, night sweats, arthralgias, myalgias, nausea, vomiting, abdominal cramps, and diarrhea. Physical examination may find generalized lymphadenopathy, splenomegally, a maculopapular rash, or pharyngeal injection.[22] Most neurological symptoms first appear with the acute generalized illness, but they may be the initial presentation shortly after HIV infection or coincident with seroconversion.[23] See table 1–3.

The primary CNS syndromes associated with HIV follow:

1. *Aseptic meningitis*—acute or subacute with chronic headaches.
2. *Vacuolar myelopathy*—ataxia, spastic paresis, dementia.
3. *Progressive HIV encephalopathy of childhood*—developmental and brain growth impairment with possible seizures or ataxia.
4. *Chronic HIV encephalopathy in adults*—or "AIDS dementia complex," the most common cause of chronic neurological dysfunction in HIV-infected adults.[23]

Of these, only the HIV encephalopathy syndrome will be discussed in detail. A graph of the relative frequency and timing of the major neurological manifestations of HIV infection can be seen in figure 1–1 from Janssen and colleagues[24].

HIV encephalopathy
Early clinical manifestations of HIV encephalopathy include cognitive symptoms (poor concentration, slowed thinking, confusion), behavioral symptoms (fatigue, depression, personality change), and motor symptoms (clumsy gait, poor handwriting, limb weakness). Even among seropositive persons considerable affective response—anxiety and depression—is present. Hong and co-workers reported that 50% of 26 seropositive individuals met criteria for a diagnosis of depression and that 40% experienced major

Table 1–3. Initial neurologic presentations of HIV infection

A major symptom	Diagnosis
Headache	Acute aseptic meningitis
Behavioral change	HIV encephalopathy
Grand mal seizure	HIV encephalitis
Syncope	Autonomic neuropathy
Truncal rash	Acute herpes zoster
Limb weakness	Guillain-Barré syndrome
Myalgia	Acute myopathy
Sleep disorder	Major depression
Hallucinations	Acute psychosis

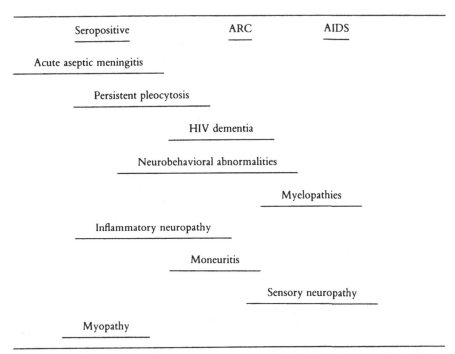

Figure 1–1. HIV-related neurological diseases. "Graph of the relative frequency (vertical axis) and timing of the major neurologic manifestations of HIV-1 infection. This graph is a rough schematic based on current knowledge and can serve as a general guide only." (Source: Janssen et al.[24])

depression.[25] Interestingly, affective response is greater among those with ARC than with AIDS.[26] Late manifestations of HIV encephalopathy are those of frank dementia: mutism, seizures, and pyramidal tract signs.[27] On the one hand, clinicians are increasingly aware of the possibility of missing the subtle signs of HIV infection; on the other hand, as McAllister and Harrison stated, "There is a real hazard that treatable options such as depression or metabolic derangement will be missed because of the growing enthusiasm for diagnosing AIDS dementia."[28] Table 1–4 lists the diagnostic features of HIV encephalopathy.

Changes in brain electrical activity—either on EEG or clinically manifested as seizures—occur in HIV-positive persons and those with ARC or AIDS. In a recent study Norcross-Nechay and colleagues concluded that "EEG background slowing is present in the majority of HIV-positive patients even when no HIV encephalopathy is suspected clinically."[29] Seizures may be the presenting symptom of HIV infection,[30] and according to a study by Wong and co-workers, focal brain pathology is not present in the majority of patients with HIV infection and seizures.[31]

Cerebrospinal fluid (CSF) abnormalities occurring after HIV infection

Table 1-4. HIV encephalopathy: Diagnostic features

Symptoms	Cognitive: confusion, slowed thinking
	Behavioral: depression, personality change
Signs	Motor: clumsy gait, limb weakness
EEG	Background slowing
CSF	↑ Protein, mononuclear cells, IgG
CT	Subcortical brain atrophy (SBA)
MRI	SBA and periventricular demyelination

include increased protein, mononuclear cells, and IgG. Even HIV has been recovered from seropositive asymptomatic persons.[32] In the U.S. Air Force, all active duty personnel are screened for HIV. A study by Appleman et al. of consecutive HIV-positive referrals disclosed 38.6% of 57 had abnormal CSF; all had neuropsychiatric testing, but only one had any neurologic finding (an abnormal magnetic resonance imaging [MRI]).[33] These and other reports suggest very early CNS involvement by HIV.[34] Portegies et al. recently indicated that HIV-1 antigen expression in the CSF is not useful in predicting neurological deterioration.[35]

Computed tomography (CT) and MRI are helpful in diagnosis. CT reveals subcortical brain atrophy, and MRI reveals atrophy and demyelinative lesions in the periventricular white matter. As disease progresses past the asymptomatic stage, demyelination and cell reactions become more prominent. Both CT and MRI may be insensitive early in the disease,[36] although they may detect pathology before the onset of clinical symptoms.[37]

In summary, HIV infection appears to be accompanied by an antigenemia, at which time the CNS may be seeded. The virus gains access to the CSF shortly after, with resultant protein and cellular abnormalities. In several weeks, with seroconversion, aseptic meningitis, grand mal seizures, or acute polyneuropathy may occur. Encephalopathy may be present very early and appears to worsen with increasing immunosuppression. Moreover, opportunistic organisms increasingly infect the host, whose ability to defend itself is severely compromised. The result is an overwhelmed host with major system deterioration.

Pathogenesis of HIV encephalopathy

HIV encephalopathy is problematic for a number of reasons: It can be the initial presentation of HIV;[37] the subtle cognitive and behavioral changes make early diagnosis difficult;[27] there is a high prevalence of neuropsychologic involvement in asymptomatic HIV-positive individuals;[38] and it may mimic diverse psychiatric illnesses.[39] Moreover, patients with moderate or severe dementia may have, although not commonly, only subtle histopathologic findings;[40] azidothymidine, an inhibitor of HIV replication, has produced dramatic improvement in adults[41] and children,[42] who have also improved with gammaglobulin alone.[43] Finally, HIV encephalopathy is so common. In

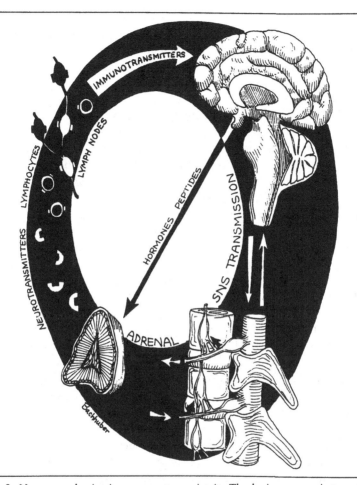

Figure 1–2. Nervous-endocrine-immune systems circuit. The brain communicates with the endocrine system anatomically via the spinal cord and the sympathetic nervous system (SNS). It also communicates with endocrine glands via hormones and peptides. The adrenal gland communicates via neurotransmitters with lymphocytes and lymph nodes, which communicate with the brain.

one study 90% of those who had progressed to ARC or AIDS had pathologic evidence of subacute encephalitis at autopsy.[15]

Price and colleagues postulated that HIV has low neurovirulence as long as "immune defenses restrict its replication and spread."[44] Support for this premise comes from the field of psychoneuroimmunology. The demonstrated interrelationship of the immune, endocrine, and central nervous systems, based on shared peptides, predicts that immune system dysfunction has neuropsychiatric ramifications.[45] Alteration in immune function associated with depression had been previously demonstrated in patients without HIV infection.[46] Further, drugs used to treat depression (monoamine oxidase inhibitors and lithium carbonate) have immunomodulatory effects.[47] A nervous-endocrine-immune systems circuit, demonstrating the proposed interaction of these systems, and described in detail in the chapter 2, is depicted in figure 1–2. The preceding discussion suggests that neuronal dysfunction, not neuronal death, is the most common cause of HIV neurological symptomatology.

Control of HIV infection, via antiviral therapy, would come best from "enhanced immune response in the host," reported Levy and Ziegler.[48] Antiviral activity, they continued, "should last as long as other conditions in which the immune response keeps viruses 'in check' in the body. A normal life span should then be expected for those HIV-infected individuals whose immune systems have learned to handle and maintain effective responses against the virus." This hypothesis sees AIDS as an opportunistic infection. Given this view, we may ask: Is the host immunocompromised prior to infection? Does the host at times participate with the virus in producing the immunocompromised state? Does this state then perpetuate and enhance viral activity? And, is this a reversible state by means other than exogenous anti-HIV therapy?

PERIPHERAL NERVOUS SYSTEM

Subclinical evidence of peripheral neuropathy has been found in 50%—90% of all patients with AIDS.[49] Four basic pathologic processes appear to result in four HIV disorders of the peripheral nervous system: immune-mediated neuropathy, vasculitic neuropathy, dying-back neuropathy, and ischemic neuropathy. They arise as though "disease-stage specific."[50] See table 1–5. The first disorder occurs early on, at the time of seroconversion in the asymptomatic individual. This inflammatory demyelinating polyneuropathy can be either acute (Guillain-Barré syndrome—GBS) or chronic (chronic relapsing inflammatory demyelinating polyneuropathy—CRIP).[51] The second disorder, Multiple mononeuropathy (MM), occurs primarily in those with ARC.[52] The third and most common disorder, predominantly sensory neuropathy (PSN), is found in those with AIDS and with later-stage ARC.[53] The fourth disorder, herpes zoster virus (HZ) and its common sequela post-herpetic neuralgia (PHN), may be the initial manifestation of HIV[54] or appear in those with ARC or AIDS.[55]

Chapter 6 presents an expanded consideration of the Guillain-Barré syndrome, predominantly sensory neuropathy, and herpes zoster in the individual with HIV infection, since they parallel conditions, in non-HIV patients, now treated by anesthesiologists with subcutaneous, epidural, and sympathetic local anesthetic nerve blocks to produce analgesia.

AUTONOMIC NERVOUS SYSTEM

In 1987 several reports noted the association of autonomic neuropathy and HIV infection.[56–58] Craddock and colleagues[56] reported syncopal episodes in

Table 1–5. Peripheral nervous system: Pathologic Processes

1. Immune-mediated	Guillain-Barré syndrome/chronic relapsing inflammatory polyneuropathy
2. Vasculitic neuropathy	Multiple mononeuropathy
3. Dying-back neuropathy	Predominantly sensory neuropathy
4. Ischemic neuropathy	Herpes zoster

Table 1–6. Ewing's provocative tests of the ANS

1. Measurement of the heart rate response to Valsalva maneuver
2. The heart rate (RR interval) variation during deep breathing
3. The immediate heart rate response to standing (30/15 RR ratio)
4. The blood pressure response to standing (fall in systolic BP)
5. The blood pressure response to sustained handgrip (increase in diastolic BP)

Source: Ewing.[91]

five patients with AIDS after fine-needle aspiration of the lung. One patient died. Subsequently, they found that in one of these individuals, and in four others, the autonomic nervous system (ANS) was abnormal. Ewing's provocative tests of the autonomic nervous system were used to assess these patients;[59] see table 1–6. All five patients assessed had abnormalities in at least two of the three heart rate tests, a sign of definite autonomic neuropathy. Three had severe autonomic neuropathy: abnormality in all three heart rate tests and one blood pressure test.

Although these syncopal episodes occurred after bradycardia and hypotension, they are similar to episodes described after respiratory arrest in patients with diabetic autonomic neuropathy. The induction of general, spinal, and epidural anesthesia, along with other procedures, has resulted in cardiorespiratory arrest in patients with and without diabetes.[60–62]

Craddock and colleagues and others[56, 63] suggested that autonomic neuropathy may be present in those with HIV infection, before AIDS develops. Craddock et al. also proposed that "the hitherto unexplained clinical features of AIDS, such as diarrhea, disordered sweating, and impotence, may be the result of underlying autonomic dysfunction."[56]

Confalonieri et al.[64] studied 29 HIV-positive intravenous drug abusers (IVDAs) and measured their circulating immune complexes (CIC). They found that 65% had autonomic nervous system involvement (24% severe) and concluded its severity is related to circulating immune complex increase (IgG and Clq) and not to clinical severity or immunologic failure. These researchers stated that this study supports the hypothesis of an immune etiopathology of autonomic nervous system involvement.[64]

NEUROMUSCULAR SYSTEM

Polymyositis occurs in people with HIV infection: seropositive, ARC, and

AIDS. Such people present with proximal muscle weakness and an elevated creatinine kinase.[65] The most common type of myopathy is an inflammatory myopathy, with perivascular or interstitial infiltrates or myofibril necrosis.[66] Involvement may be primary HIV, secondary to coinfection with another virus, or secondary to abnormal immunoregulation.[23] Lange et al. stated that, except for the neuromuscular junction, every part of the neuromuscular system seems vulnerable to HIV infection.[67]

CONCLUSION

Human immunodeficiency virus infection covers a wide spectrum of illness, involving apparently healthy asymptomatic people to those in the advanced state of AIDS. The viral RNA contains genes that regulate HIV synthesis, determine virus infectivity, and down-regulate HIV replication. Variation in gene activity, host immune defense, and many other cofactors determine the rapidity and progression of the disease.

That the CNS is infected early has confused the separation of psychological and neurological presentations; in fact, the two are likely intertwined. Immunosuppression compounds the problem; for example, neurologic disease can be either a direct result of HIV or a direct or indirect result of HIV immunosuppression. The depression seen with HIV encephalopathy is a premier example of the difficulty in sorting out diagnosis and treatment.

Since peripheral nervous system disorders are common among those with HIV infection, and anesthesiologists have demonstrated benefit to other people with neural blockade procedures, it is relevant to extend these treatment modalities to those with HIV infection. Both the relief of pain and the aid in treatment or resolution of the neurologic symptoms magnify the benefit for people in whom increasing pain and neurologic symptomatology can exacerbate their illness. Treatment for these syndromes will be detailed in chapter 6.

NOTE

This chapter appears as a portion of a larger chapter by this author in the second edition of *Practical Management of Pain*, edited by P. Prithvi Raj, Yearbook Medical Publishers, Chicago.

REFERENCES

1. Gallo RC, Wong-Staal F: A human T-lymphotrophic retrovirus (HTLV-III) as the cause of the acquired immune deficiency syndrome. Ann Intern Med 103:679–689, 1985.
2. Coffin J, Haase A, Levy JA, et al: Human immunodeficiency viruses (letter). Science 232:697, 1986.
3. Clavel F, Geutard D, Brun-Vezinet F, et al: Isolation of a new human retrovirus from West African patients with AIDS. Science 233:343–346, 1986.
4. Ho DD, Pomerantz RJ, Kaplan JC: Pathogenesis of infection with human immunodeficiency virus. N Engl J Med 317:278–286, 1987.
5. Bowen DL, Lane HC, Fauci AS: Immunopathogenesis of the acquired immunodeficiency syndrome. Ann Int Med 103:704–709, 1985.

6. Gartner S, Markovits P, Markovitz DM, et al: The role of mononuclear phagocytes in HTLV-III/LAV infection. Science 233:215–219, 1986.
7. Haverkos HW: Factors associated with the pathogenesis of AIDS. J Infect Dis 156:251–257, 1987.
8. Pahwa S, Rahwa R, Good RA, et al: Stimulatory and inhibitory influences of human immunodeficiency virus on normal B lymphocytes. Proc Natl Acad Sci USA 83:9124–9128, 1986.
9. Saxon A, Campen V: AIDS: state of the art, spring 1988. J Allergy Clin Immunol 81(5):796–802, 1988.
10. Update: Acquired immunodeficiency syndrome (AIDS)—United States. MMWR 32:688–691, 1984.
11. Goedert JJ: Testing for human immunodeficiency virus. Ann Intern Med 105:609, 1986.
12. Bredesen DE, Messing R: Neurological syndromes heralding the acquired immunodeficiency syndrome (abstract). Ann Neurol 14:141, 1983.
13. Berger JR, Moskowitz L, Fischl M, Kelley RE: Neurologic disease as the presenting manifestation of acquired immunodeficiency syndrome. South Med J 80:683–686, 1987.
14. Gabuzda DH, Hirsch MS: Neurologic manifestations of infection with human immunodeficiency virus. Ann Intern Med 107:383–391, 1987.
15. de la Monte SM, Ho DD, Schooley RT, et al: Subacute encephalomyelitis of AIDS and its relation to HTLV-III infection. Neurology 37:562–569, 1987.
16. Berger Jr: The neurological complications of HIV infection. Acta Neur Scand 116(S):40–76, 1988.
17. Pert CB, Smith CC, Ruff MR, Hill JM: AIDS and its dementia as a neuropeptide disorder: Role of VIP receptor blockade by human immunodeficiency virus envelope. Ann Neurol 23(S):71–73, 1988.
18. Klatzman D, Barre-Sinoussi F, Nugeyre M, et al: Selective trophism of lymphadenopathy-associated virus (LAV) for helper-inducer T-lymphocytes. Science 225:59–62, 1984.
19. Wiley CA, Schrier RD, Nelson JA, et al: Cellular localization of the AIDS retrovirus infection within the brains of acquired immune deficiency syndrome patients. Proc Natl Acad Sci USA 83:7089–7093, 1986.
20. Cheng-Mayer C, Levy JA: Distinct biologic and serologic properties of HIV isolates from the brain. Ann Neurol 23(S):58–61, 1988.
21. Ranki A, Vallf SL, Krohn M, et al: Long latency precedes overt seroconversion in sexually transmitted immunodeficiency-virus infection. Lancet 2:589–593, 1987.
22. Ho DD, Sarngadharan MG, Resnick L, et al: Primary human T-lymphotrophic virus type III infection. Ann Intern Med 103:880–883, 1985.
23. Dalakas M, Wichman A, Sever J: AIDS and the nervous system. JAMA 261(16):2396–2399, 1989.
24. Janssen RS, Cornblath DR, Epstein LG, et al: Human immunodeficiency virus (HIV) infection and the nervous system: Report from the American Academy of Neurology AIDS Task Force. Neurology 39:119–122, 1989.
25. Hong BA, Rice J, Brookshire D, Guedet P: Diagnosis of depression in HIV infected individuals. Vth International Conference on AIDS, Montreal, Abs# MBP383, 1989.
26. Holland JC, Toss S: The psychosocial and neuropsychiatric sequelae of the immunodeficiency syndrome and related disorders. Ann Intern Med 103:760–764, 1985.
27. Price RW, Sidtis J, Rosenblum M: The AIDS dementia complex: Some current questions. Ann Neurol 23(S):23–33, 1988.
28. McAllister RH, Harrison MJ: HIV and the nervous system. BR J Hosp Med 40(1):21–26, 1988.
29. Norcross-Nechay K, Boruchi MJ, Boruchi SJ, Pollard RJ: Definite EEG background changes occur early in HIV-positive patients. Neurology 39(S):361, 1989.
30. Kaku DA, Holtzman DM, So YT: Seizures and AIDS: An analysis of 100 patients. Neurology 39(S):362, 1989.
31. Wong MC, Suite ND, Labar DR: Seizures in HIV infection. Neurology 39(S):362, 1989.
32. Chiodi F, Asjo B, Fenyo EM: Isolation of human immunodeficiency virus from cerebrospinal fluid of antibody-positive virus carrier without neurological symptoms. Lancet 2:1276–1277, 1986.
33. Appleman ME, Marshall DW, Brey RL, et al: Cerebrospinal fluid abnormalities in patients

without AIDS who are seropositive for the human immunodeficiency virus. J Infect Dis 158(1):193–199, 1988.

34. Hollander H: Cerebrospinal fluid normalities and abnormalities in individuals infected with human immunodeficiency virus. J Infect Dis, 158(4):855–858, 1988.

35. Portegies P, Epstein LG, Hung STA, et al: Human immunodeficiency virus type 1 antigen in cerebrospinal fluid. Arch Neurol 46:261–264, 1989.

36. Post MJ, Sheldon JJ, Hensley GT, et al: Central nervous system disease in acquired immunodeficiency syndrome: Prospective correlation using CT, MR imaging and pathologic studies. Radiology 158:141–148, 1986.

37. Navia BA, Price RW: AIDS dementia complex as the presenting or sole manifestation of HIV infection. Arch Neurol 44:65–72, 1987.

38. Grant I, Atkinson JH, Hesselink JR, et al: Evidence for early central nervous system involvement in the acquired immunodeficiency syndrome (AIDS) and other human immunodeficiency virus (HIV) infections: Studies with neuropsychologic testing and magnetic resonance imaging. Ann Intern Med 107:828–836, 1987.

39. Resnick L, DiMarzo-Veronesa F, Schupbach J, et al: Intra-blood-brain-barrier synthesis of HTLV-III specific IgG in patients with neurologic symptoms associated with AIDS or AIDS-related complex. N Engl J Med 313:1498–1504, 1985.

40. Petito CK: Review of central nervous system pathology in human immunodeficiency virus infection. Ann Neurol 23(S):54–57, 1988.

41. Yarchoan R, Brouwers P, Spitzer AR, et al: Response of human immunodeficiency-virus-associated neurological disease to 3'-azido-3'deoxythymidine. Lancet 1:132–135, 1987.

42. Matthies J, Walker LA, Watson JG, Bird AG: AIDS encephalopathy with response to treatment. Arch Dis Child 63:545–547, 1988.

43. Gupta A, Novick BE, Rubenstein A: Restoration of supressor T cell functions in children with AIDS following gammaglobulin treatment. Am J Dis Child 140:143–146, 1986.

44. Price RW, Brew B, Sidtis J, et al: The brain in AIDS: Central nervous system HIV-1 infection and AIDS dementia complex. Science 239:586–592, 1988.

45. Blalock JE, McMenamin DH, Smith EM: Peptide hormones shared by the neuroendocrine and immunologic systems. J Immunol 135:858s–861s, 1985.

46. Lieb J: Remission off rheumatoid arthritis and other disorders of immunity in patients taking monoamine oxidase inhibitors. Int J Immunopharmacol 5:353–357, 1983.

47. Verma DS, Spitzer G, Gutterman JU: Human leukocyte interferon mediated granulopoietic differentiation arrest and its abrogation by lithium carbonate. Amer J Hematol, 12:39–46, 1982.

48. Levy JA, Ziegler JL: Acquired immune deficiency syndrome (AIDS) is an opportunistic infection and Kaposi's sarcoma results from secondary immune stimulation. Lancet 2:78–81, 1983.

49. De la Monte SM, Gabuzda DH, Ho DD, et al: Peripheral neuropathy in the acquired immune deficiency syndrome (abstract). Lab Invest 56:17, 1987.

50. Cornblath DR, McArthur JC: Predominantly sensory neuropathy in patients with AIDS and AIDS-related complex. Neurology 38:794–796, 1988.

51. Cornblath DR, McArthur JC, Kennedy PG, et al: Inflammatory demyelinating peripheral neuropathies associated with human T-cell lymphotrophic virus type III infection. Ann Neurol 21:32–40, 1987.

52. Cornblath DR, McArthur JC, Griffin JW: The spectrum of peripheral neuropathies in HTLV-III infection. Muscle Nerve 9(S):76, 1986.

53. Levy RM, Bredesen DE, Rosenblum ML: Neurological manifestations of the acquired immunodeficiency syndrome: Experience at UCSF and review of the literature. J Neurosur 62:475–495, 1985.

54. Friedman-Kien AE, Lafleur FL, Gendler E, Hennessey NP: Herpes zoster: A possible early clinical sign for development of acquired immunodeficiency syndrome in high-risk individuals. J Am Acad Dermatol, 14:1023–1028, 1986.

55. Wilkerson MG, Jordan WP, Kerkering TM: Herpes zoster as a sign of AIDS-related complex. American Family Physician 36(4):233–235, 1987.

56. Craddock C, Bull R, Pasvol, et al: Cardiorespiratory arrest and autonomic neuropathy in AIDS. Lancet 4:16–18, 1987.

57. Lin-Greenberger A, Taneja-Uppal N: Dysautonomia and infection with the human immunodeficiency virus. Ann Intern Med 106:167, 1987.

58. Miller RF, Semple SJ: Autonomic neuropathy in AIDS. Lancet 2:343–344, 1987.
59. Ewing DJ, Clarke BF: Autonomic neuropathy: Its diagnosis and prognosis. Clin Endocrinol Metab 15:855–888, 1986.
60. Page MMcB, Watkins PJ: Cardiorespiratory arrest and diabetic autonomic neuropathy. Lancet 1:14–16, 1978.
61. Wetstone DL, Wong KC: Sinus bradycardia and asystole during spinal anesthesia. Anesthesiology 41:87–89, 1974.
62. Caplan RA, Ward RJ, Posner BA, Cheney FW: Unexpected cardiac arrest during spinal anesthesia: A closed claims analysis of predisposing factors. Anesthesiology 68:5–11, 1988.
63. Villa A, Foresti V, Confalonieri F: Autonomic neuropathy and HIV infection. Lancet 8564:915, 1987.
64. Confalonieri F, Villa A, Cruccu V, et al: Possible pathogenetic role of immune complexes in HIV-related autonomic neuropathy. Vth International Conference on AIDS, Abs# TBP 191, 447, Montreal, 1989.
65. Cornblath, DR: Treatment of the neuromuscular complications of human immunodeficiency virus infection. Ann Neurol 23(S):88–91, 1988.
66. Dalakas MC, Pezeshkpour GH: Neuromuscular diseases associated with human immunodeficiency virus infection. Ann Neurol 23(S):38–48, 1988.
67. Lange DJ, Britton CB, Younger DS, Hays AP: The neuromuscular manifestations of human immunodeficiency virus infections. Arch Neurol 45:1084–1088, 1988.

2. PSYCHONEUROIMMUNOLOGY AND AIDS

SANFORD I. COHEN AND SUSAN BLUMENTHAUL

WHAT IS PSYCHONEUROIMMUNOLOGY?

Psychoneuroimmunology (PNI) studies the psychological influences in immune function, psychosocial variables in disease and healing, experimental immune conditioning of animals, and biological mechanisms underlying these processes. The field of psychoneuroimmunology has only begun to emerge as a distinct discipline in the past decade, although studies in this area have been underway since the 1960s. At that time the major hypothesis was that life stress through PNI links could exert an immunosuppressive influence.[1]

Today, however, PNI is concerned with the complex bidirectional interactions between the central nervous system (mediating both psychic and biologic processes) and the immune system. Despite its youth, the field is tackling many of the important issues in understanding the links between mind and body. As is often the case with a new discipline, psychoneuroimmunology research is beginning to address in proper scientific terms questions considered too complex or even "unscientific" to be considered previously. This progress is due in part to the coalescing of concerns and methodologies of the fields forming psychoneuroimmunology to modify and broaden the experimental designs of studies. This attempt to explore directly the links among mind, brain, and immune function may thus open the door to understanding some of the oldest questions posed by man but now facilitated by modern concepts and technologies.

Psychoneuroimmunology reinforces the view that all disease is multifactorial and biopsychosocial in cause, onset, and course—the result of interrelationships among specific etiologic factors (such as microbes, carcinogens, and genetic, endocrine, immune, emotional, and behavioral). The immune system is regulated at cellular, hormonal, and central nervous system levels, and different principles may be required to understand how it behaves at these levels. The immune system is an interactive, interregulatory network held in delicate balance by complex relationships among cell sets. Cunningham coined the phrase *gestalt immunology* to emphasize the need for a new appreciation of the holistic aspects of how this immune network functions.[2,3] Cunningham's thesis is that many immune functions, such as control, may be impossible to understand if we rely entirely on the "classical" scientific method of reducing the system to its simplest elements and predicting the behavior of the whole from the properties of the parts. Cunningham argued that if we think of the immune system as a network, a fresh understanding of its operation might be gained. Given the interrelationships between the immune and nervous systems, one also wonders whether more direct conceptual cross-fertilization between immunology and the neurosciences (i.e., in such related endeavors as artificial intelligence research) might not also yield unexpected advances in our understanding of these complex, intertwined systems.[4]

BRIEF HISTORICAL REVIEW OF PSYCHONEUROIMMUNOLOGY
A large number of studies in psychoneuroimmunology have emerged in the last few years as a result of an increasing interest in the mechanisms through which psychosocial stress and related emotional and mental phenomena affect physical disease. However, the connections between mind and illness have long been known to physicians and folk healers.

An interesting article written by Ishigami in 1918 dealt with the potential impact of psychological factors on infectious diseases.[5] This paper was the forerunner of concepts that would be reported extensively a half century later. Other studies reported an increased susceptibility to viral infections,[6] coxsackievirus,[7] and polio in animals exposed to stress.[8] Later articles by Imboden et al. on influenza,[9] by Meyer and Haggerty on streptococcal infections,[10] and by Solomon and Moos[11] on rheumatoid arthritis suggest how infectious and immune-related diseases may be influenced by psychological states and related endocrine changes.

In the 1940s and 1950s, the influence of the pituitary-adrenal system on lymphocytes was described.[12] These early studies were efforts to suggest that stress-related hormonal responses might modify lymphocytic functions. Studies of the influence of hormones on various immune functions were largely concerned with the impact of acute systemic stress on immune responsiveness as mediated by the activation of the pituitary-adrenal system.[13] This led to explorations of the network of immune neuroendocrine interactions and the notion of afferent and efferent CNS pathways between the immune and endocrine systems.[14] Antigenic stimulation was described as changing the electrical activity of the hypothalamus and causing major endocrine responses that had implications for the development and maintenance of immunoregulation and immunospecificity.[14,15] Papers on neuroimmunomodulation, from the late 1950s and early 1960s, represent some of the earliest efforts to study the relation of hypothalamic functions in immunogenesis, in particular, antigen–antibody reactions.[16–19] These research studies of the neurophysiological mechanisms affecting the immune system were undertaken prior to widespread interest in this field in the United States. In the late 1960s and 1970s, studies described the effects of antibrain antibodies, the regulatory influences of the immune system on brain activity,[20] and immunoregulation mediated by the sympathetic nervous system.[21,22] These contributions were followed by the work of Bartrop et al. on the effects of bereavement[23] and by Kasl et al.'s article on psychosocial factors in the development of infectious mononucleosis.[24] The latter study was one of the few prospective investigations in this particular field.

The relationship between the immune system and mental illness has been of interest. Articles by Dameshek[25] and by Fessel and Hiratu-Hiki[26] focused on changes in white blood cells in schizophrenia. Studies by Heath,[27] Solomon,[28] and Vartanian[29] implicated antibodies resulting from acute immune reactions to brain tissue as possible causes of schizophrenia.

Early studies on the relationship of behavior and immune function initially focused on the effects of exposure to experimental stress. Two pioneering articles by G. Solomon dealt with the effects of early life experiences on immune function and on the effect of stress on antibody responses in rats.[30,31] The importance of these contributions was not recognized until recently. An early attempt to identify the mechanisms through which life events and psychological reactions may affect the immune system appeared in a 1960 article by Soviet authors Dohan and Krylov.[32] A 1975 article by Ader and Cohen provides an experimental basis for these conditional reflex mechanisms.[33]

Several contemporary researchers tried to piece these results together into a coherent picture—for example *Psychoneuroimmunology*, a volume edited by Robert Ader of the University of Rochester.[34] It was followed by *Mind and Immunity*, edited by Drs. Steven Locke and Mady Hornig-Rohan.[35] This volume is a compendium of over 1,450 bibliographic citations and abstracts from 1976 to 1983 on "behavioral immunology." In 1985 Locke et al. published a collection of articles representing contributions to psychoneuroimmunology, some of which have been mentioned in this section.[36]

NEUROIMMUNOMODULATION: THE BRAIN-IMMUNE SYSTEM LINK

Spector and Korneva used the term *neuroimmunomodulation* to describe the continuous interactions among the nervous, endocrine, and immune systems that mediate psychoimmunological phenomena.[37] Many early studies in this area were conducted by Soviet and Eastern European investigators and focused on the mechanisms through which brain centers, particularly the hypothalamus, modulate immunity.[38]

A number of lesion studies have shown that destroying parts of the hypothalamus results in measurable effects on immune responses. Stein and colleagues showed that destroying the anterior (but not the posterior) portion of the hypothalamus in guinea pigs protected them against an ordinarily fatal immune response called lethal anaphylactic shock, reduced antibody responses to a foreign substance, and depressed the delayed hypersensitivity reaction to other immune challenges.[39] Roszman et al. reported that hypothalamic lesions suppressed measures of immunity, such as lymphocyte responsivity and natural killer cell activity.[40] Their research also indicated that lesions in the amygdala and hippocampus enhance the responsivity of lymphocytes in animals. Stein et al. concluded that there is no single mediating factor.[39] Various processes, including the autonomic nervous system and neuroendocrine activity, may participate. Emerging evidence affirms a role for both of these pathways.

In review of the research findings in this area, Gorman and Locke found experimental evidence that the nervous, endocrine, and immune systems circuit are highly integrated, routinely communicate with one another, mutually regulate various aspects of each other's responsiveness, and together contribute to the organism's homeostasis.[41] In this article, they identified a wide range of biological links, including the following:

1. Direct neuronal connections between the nervous and immune systems involve innervation of immune organs by nerve endings.
2. Cell-surface receptors on immune cells have been found for neuropeptides, neurotransmitters, and hormones. A variety of intercellular "communication" molecules shared by the immune and neuroendocrine system have been identified. CNS cells have been found to produce interleukin, and immune cells to produce neuropeptides.
3. Neurotransmitters, neuropeptides, neurohormones, and the trophic hormones under their control have been noted to influence the function of immune cells, both in vitro and in vivo. For example, immunity has been suppressed or enhanced by opioids, neuropeptides, adrenal and sex steroids, trophic hormones (LH, FSH, and GH), and neurotransmitters (epinephrine, norepinephrine, and serotonin).
4. Some immune hormones and peptides can influence nervous system functions. The firing rate of hypothalamic neurons can be altered during immune responses. Further, thymosin peptides, interleukins, and other immune cell products can influence hypothalamic-pituitary activity.
5. Various measures of immune function can be altered by experimental manipulations of the nervous system. Immune functions can be suppressed or enhanced by discrete limbic or hypothalamic lesions or electric stimulation, as well as by drugs that influence the CNS.

6. Immunoregulatory circuits exist that appear to operate via the hypothalamus and the neuroendocrine system. Immune cells have been reported to secrete factors that inform the CNS of factors that affect immune response.
7. Immunologic abnormalities have been reported in some individuals with psychiatric symptoms.
8. The presence of behavioral, emotional, and neurologic abnormalities have been noted in some individuals with immunologic symptoms. For example, a schizophrenic-like psychosis has been known to accompany some cases of systemic lupus erythematosus (SLE) and abate when SLE is treated.

Recent work has focused on possible biological pathways linking CNS function and host risk, including bidirectional feedback loops between endocrine and immune responsiveness. For example, a report by Besedovsky and colleagues presented evidence for an immunoregulatory feedback network between interleukin-1 (IL-1), a pyrogenic (fever-inducing) protein produced predominantly by stimulated macrophages and monocytes, and glucocorticoid hormones.[42]

It is well known, for example, that glucocorticoids can interfere with several essential steps in the immune response. Besedovsky and co-workers have shown that glucocorticoids can block IL-1 production by macrophages and can also inhibit the induction of Ia antigens necessary for antigen presentation.[42] They suggested that when IL-1 concentrations reach a critical level in the circulation, during infection or other immunological function, the pituitary-adrenal axis becomes activated and glucocorticoid blood levels thus increase. As a result, immune cell functions, including the production of cytokines such as IL-1, become down-regulated. This endocrine response reflects the existence of a feedback circuit involving products of immunocompetent cells, such as IL-1, and the pituitary-adrenal axis. Such glucocorticoid-associated immunoregulatory mechanisms may act as continuous surveillance of immunological cells and activity.[42]

In summary, the brain and the immune system are linked by two major pathways: the autonomic nervous system (ANS) and the neuroendocrine system (NES). Autonomic fibers show regional and specific innervation of both the vasculature and the parenchyma of all major lymphoid tissues, including the bone marrow, thymus, spleen, and lymph nodes. The cells and tissues of the immune system have surface, or cytoplasmic, receptors for a wide variety of neurohormones, neuropeptides, and neurotransmitters. Several lines of evidence described by Gorman and Locke support the existence of a role for the sympathetic nervous system in neural modulation of immunity.[41] Similarly, the immune and neuroendocrine systems appear to be thoroughly integrated through the expression of a shared set of hormones and a shared set of receptors for these hormones. Several afferent and efferent pathways appear to exist by which the immune and nervous systems participate in regulatory circuits. Afferent pathways allow the immune system to communicate with the nervous system and are mediated by immune cell production of neuroactive soluble factors. Efferent neuroendocrine pathways, including the hypothalamic-pituitary axis, the hypothalamic-pituitary-gonadal axis, and the pineal-melatonin and neuropeptide systems, allow the nervous system to influence immune responses. Thus, the available evidence provides some support for the theory that the immune, nervous, and endocrine systems may in fact constitute one integrated suprasystem that could, in a coordinated fashion, maintain homeostasis in the face of changing external and internal conditions.

Conditioning of the immune response

In 1975 Ader and Cohen reported that the humoral immune response can be conditioned.[33] In their study rats were injected with cyclophosphamide, a drug that suppresses immune function, at the same time they were given saccharine-flavored drinking water. Following a suitable conditioning period, the same rats were given only the saccharine-flavored drinking water. Subsequent presentation of the saccharin to the animal prevented the antibody response to sheep red blood cells. Thus their immune function was suppressed exactly as though they had been given cyclophosphamide. That the immune system can be conditioned is one of the early findings in psychoneuroimmunology. Initially, it was also one of the most controversial, for it implies that the immune system—long thought to be autonomous and free of external regulation—and the central nervous system are inextricably linked. It also suggests that the complex network of molecules and cells responsible for safeguarding our health and well-being can be shaped and reshaped by experience and by environmental stimuli.

Ader reviewed earlier studies that had suggested conditioning effects on immune function.[43] Further, Ader and Cohen's results have been both replicated and extended to other immunosuppressive agents[44,45] and a variety of conditioned stimuli. Ader's ongoing research program now seeks to clarify issues of theoretical interest with respect to conditioning as well as the applicability of conditioning to pharmacotherapeutic regimes. Can the undesirable consequences of chemotherapy, for instance, be reduced by alternating the administration of drugs with unwanted side effects with other less harmless, drugs to which the patient has been conditioned to respond?

Cellular immunity[46] and natural killer (NK) cell activity[47] have also been conditioned, and the technique has been used to prolong the lives of mice with the autoimmune disease, lupus erythematosus.[48] Gorczynski first gave mice three consecutive skin grafts from other mice and measured their immune responses to these grafts.[49] He then subjected them to a sham graft in which they experienced all of the behavioral procedures and environmental cues they had learned to associate with grafting, without any skin actually being grafted. The mice showed the same initial lymphocyte response to the sham graft as they had to the actual skin graft.

Spector reviewed the history of immune response conditioning and perspectives for its clinical applications in the prevention and treatment of human disease.[50] He pointed out that alteration of immune responses by classical Pavlovian conditioning, a form of learning most impressively demonstrating back-and-forth communication between systems, was shown not only for immunosuppression but also for enhancement of the immune functions, for example, natural killer cell activity. One provocative finding mentioned by Spector was that a multiple myeloma could be totally reversed in some mice as a result of prior conditioning.

Research on immunity and conditioning implies that the immune system is intimately connected with the central nervous system. It also suggests new approaches to studying individual differences in experience that shape the complex relationship among personality, stress, immune function, health, and disease.

STRESS AND THE IMMUNE SYSTEM

Stress research has received considerable theoretical and empirical attention. Many studies have documented an association between stressors and the onset of illness or the worsening of health. Evidence suggests that distressful situations, induced by environmental and/or psychosocial factors, may affect immune responsiveness. Various forms of "stress" modulate the immune system in different ways, either by enhancing or by inhibiting immune function. Data from both the biological and behavioral fields also suggest that stress reduction can reduce vulnerability to infection and psychological morbidity and can facilitate more adaptive coping. Over the past years there has developed a broad conceptualization of the relationship between stress and health and illness. Stressors have been noted to influence bodily functions in both health and disease. These influences are thought to be mediated biologically through the CNS and endocrine and immune systems and mediated behaviorally through coping mechanisms and social supports.

Study of the influences of stress on immunity and on disease susceptibility is complicated by a number of factors. One such factor is the difficulty in defining "stress." Research on the biological consequences of stress has produced a plethora of divergent, often vague, definitions as to what constitutes stress. The term has been used to refer to the impact of an external event, how the event is perceived, the subjective experience of distress resulting from such impact, the ability to cope with the event, the biological response, or the interaction or combination of these effects. The appearance of these multiple definitions of stress in the literature complicates a review of the effects of stressful stimuli on immune function.

Another complicating factor is the difficulty of separating the direct immunological effects of a behavioral state, such as bereavement, from the indirect immunological effects resulting from bereavement-associated changes in diet, sleep patterns, drug intake, and consumption of cigarettes or alcohol, all known to affect immune function. Some investigators eliminate many of these variables by using animal models of psychological and behavioral stress paradigms; such animal models raise different methodological issues about the measurement of "emotion" and "stress" in animals, particularly whether findings based on animal models can be extrapolated to humans.

Another major issue arises from lack of hard data about what magnitudes of immune alteration represent clinically significant abnormalities. Immunological alterations have often been found to be associated with behavioral and emotional states; however, the clinical significance of these alterations to the onset and course of human disease has not been established. Furthermore, suppression of various parameters of immune function is not always harmful, nor is enhancement always beneficial.

Research should benefit from a revision of stress concepts. It has become increasingly apparent that stress is not a specific, unitary entity. It is a convenient code word that subsumes a large variety of internal and external forces acting on the organism. Early stress researchers looked primarily at stress responses from a biological perspective, although they noted repeatedly that stress responses were influenced by psychosocial as well as biological factors.[51] Even when they finally accepted or at least considered it possible that life stress, psychological reactions, emotions, thoughts, and behavior might be legitimate factors influencing, or influenced by, body functions, they did not relinquish the mind-body dichotomy or biomedical causality model, that is, a specific cause leading to a specific effect. The inclusion of psychosocial factors as potential influences on the body seems to have required the adoption of a stress model in which stress achieved the status of a causative agent such as a bacterium, poison, or tumor. However, the stress model was, at best, a "pseudo-systems" model.

The notion of specific biological patterns associated with definable psychosocial events and emotional signals that mobilize a specific behavioral response now seems a more useful framework for understanding stress. The application of this model to studies of immune function should increase our understanding of the complex interactions between psychosocial stressors and biological functions.

PSYCHONEUROIMMUNOLOGY OF HOPELESSNESS

This section focuses on specific types of emotional response—namely, hopelessness, despair, and depression—as potentially significant influences on biological function. A number of studies have demonstrated the effects of these affective states on the onset, perpetuation, or worsening of a wide range of physical illnesses. The psychoneuroimmunology of hopelessness may be particularly relevant to the course of AIDS infection and is discussed in the next section.

Pertinent findings from animal studies have indicated that the effects of loss, separation, or the inability to master or control the environment significantly affect immune function. Experiments have shown that animals exposed to conditions they cannot control may be vulnerable to premature death as well as to a variety of biological changes.[52] There have also been a number of reports of animals dying suddenly of unknown causes in situations such as captivity or upon being transferred from a familiar to unfamiliar locale. In primates, deaths have occurred after the mate had died, and sudden death has been observed in primates separated from their mothers or after experiencing what appear to be meaningful losses.[53]

In most animal studies, sudden death occurred after exposure to conditions similar to human psychosocial stressors (threatening situations). Death seemed related to ventricular arrhythmias associated with sympathetic nervous system overstimulation.[54,55] A few studies reported cardiac slowing and arrest, associated with massive vagal discharge.[56-59]

Other studies have reported that psychosocial, environmental, and mechanical stressors produce increases in plasma adrenal corticoids and other hormones through well-described neuroendocrine pathways. These hormonal changes are often accompanied by alterations in immune function that heighten vulnerability to the action of latent oncologic viruses and other incipient pathological processes normally held in check by an intact immunologic apparatus.[60]

In some experiments, animals were exposed to unpredictable and inescapable shock. The response of these animals has been called "learned helplessness" and is believed by some investigators to be an excellent animal model for human depression.[61] These helpless animals have shown decreased T-cell number and function.[62] It was noted that the experimental conditions suppressed the stimulation of lymphocytes in adrenalectomized animals. Hence, stress-related adrenal secretion of corticosteroids or catecholamines is not required for stress-induced suppression of lymphocyte stimulation by T-cell mitogen in the rats.[63]

In studies of learned helplessness, Post indicated that the ability to cope with a noxious stimulus can alter brain norepinephrine.[64] If an animal is subjected to shock from which it can escape, there is little effect on levels of brain or plasma norepinephrine. By contrast, a yoked animal, unable to escape, that receives a shock of equal intensity and duration will show depletion in norepinephrine. Returning the animal to the environment in which it was originally shocked is sufficient to reproduce some of the original biochemical depletion of neurotransmitter.[65]

Stein studied the effect of bereavement in men whose wives had advanced cancer.[63,66] Findings included the decreased ability of their lymphocytes to respond to an activating agent in the month or two after their wives' death. Suppression of mitogen-induced lymphocyte stimulation appeared to be a direct consequence of bereavement.

Even though the death of a spouse is considered one of the most stressful human experiences, the power of this loss to enhance susceptibility to physical illness remains controversial. Epidemiologic studies suggest that mortality is higher among older widowers. The data for widows, however, are equivocal. Such studies suggest that women may be more resistant than men to the adverse health consequences of bereavement. However, Irwin and colleagues compared natural killer cell activity (a component of the immune surveillance system) in women whose husbands had recently died with that found in age-matched controls who had not experienced recent adverse life events.[67] Bereaved women had significantly lower natural killer (NK) cell activity than women whose husbands were healthy. In a second study depressive symptoms and NK activity were measured longitudinally in women before and after the death of their husbands. The results suggested that depression symptoms and not merely the death of the spouse are related to a reduction in NK activity during bereavement. Changes in the number and ratio of T cells in these women were within the normal range and do not necessarily have clinical significance. Although the pattern of changes in immune function was related to the intensity of depression symptoms, the authors stated that their findings did not necessarily generalize to patients suffering from depressive disorders. The subjects in this study were undergoing major life changes. The NK-cell suppression could be mediated by cortisol and norepinephrine elevation, which has been reported in the plasma of persons undergoing distressing life experiences.

Since depression is one consequence of bereavement, Stein decided to examine the lymphocyte responses in patients hospitalized with severe depressive disorder.[63] He found these also to be suppressed. Lymphocyte stimulation by PHA, con A, and PMW and the number of T and B cells were significantly lower for hospitalized depressed patients. The authors concluded that functional activity of the lymphocyte as well as the number of competent immune cells are decreased in clinically depressed patients.

Evidence for anatomic and chemical connections between the CNS and immune system has been accumulating. Work by Stein and colleagues and others has shown that animals with lesions of the anterior but not the posterior hypothalamus have reduced cellular and antibody-mediated immune responses to antigenic substances.[39] Life events causing psychological distress may produce immune suppression via a number of pathways; for example, CRF may trigger release of ACTH, which then stimulates the release of corticosterone and leads to suppression of immune function. Corticosterones suppress the number of lymphocytes and mitogen response. Increased HPA activity is often found in major depressive disorders. Pert[68] and Ruff[69] and their colleagues reported that animals that are made to feel helpless have macrophages that move more sluggishly than usual, probably as a result of changes in neuropeptides. These findings may help to explain why patients who feel hopeless have poorer health outcomes than those who remain optimistic. Pert suggested that neuropeptides may be a key biochemical unit of emotion since they appear in such high concentrations in the limbic system.

Additionally, it appears that the CNS and the immune system may communicate directly through specific nerve connections. Bullock reported ANS fibers that go directly to the thymus where T cells mature.[70] Recent work has also suggested that the right and left neocortex have different effects on the immune system.[71] The left cortex seems to be involved in regulating activity of the immune system, especially the activities of T cells with lesions of the left cortex that result in some T-cell dysfunction. In humans it is possible that right-brain dominance may be similar to decreasing left-brain function. The right hemisphere may be involved in the processing of negative emotions, especially depression. The point here is that altering the function of a specific area of the central nervous system may change the responsivity of the immune system, which in turn can influence resistance to infection or possibly the growth of cancer cells.

Not only can the nervous system influence immune responses, but more recent work shows immune responses can alter nerve cell activity. The cells of the immune system may function in a sensory capacity by relaying signals to the brain about stimuli such as invading pathogens.[72-74] In this way, the immune system communicates back to the hypothalamus and the autonomic and endocrine systems via substances produced by immune cells that have been called "immunotransmitters."[75]

PSYCHONEUROIMMUNOLOGICAL INFLUENCES ON AIDS

The acquired immunodeficiency syndrome (AIDS) is a major public health problem today that can be studied from a psychoneuroimmunological frame of reference.[76] It is a fatal, devastating, and incurable illness that already has had an unprecedented impact on the physical and mental health of our society. The Centers for Disease Control (CDC) estimate that between 1.5 and 2.0 million persons in the United States are infected with the human immunodeficiency virus (HIV), a retrovirus that is the etiologic agent of AIDS. To date (1989) there have been over 100,000 diagnosed cases of AIDS, more than half of whom have died. AIDS is currently the number one killer of young people between 25 and 34 in New York City. The "incubation period" of the disease can be long and varied, reportedly up to seven years.

Acquired immunodeficiency syndrome is characterized by a profound disturbance in the immune system in which the retrovirus enters and destroys key white blood cells (the T lymphocytes), thereby crippling a person's ability to fight off life-threatening illnesses, such as Pneumocystis carinii pneumonia and certain types of cancers. The virus may also enter other types of cells, such as brain cells and macrophages.

Because behavior is intimately involved with a number of key aspects of AIDS, the adoption of a biopsychosocial approach to the illness is a matter of vital practical importance. Volitional behaviors responsible for transmitting the illness are drug-using and high-risk sexual practices. Prevention of AIDS is currently entirely dependent on altering these behaviors. Additionally, the overwhelming realities of the disease and the response of family, friends, society, and health care institutions lead many patients to feel that they have lost control of their lives and that they are at the mercy of a community that wants them isolated. This loss of mastery in one's life, the isolation, and the stigmatization leads to a sense of despair, helplessness, and hopelessness that is both tragic and devastating. There are also profound psychological consequences of AIDS, including depression and anxiety. These problems may be worsened by direct invasion of the brain by HIV or from CNS infections associated with opportunistic infections (e.g., cryptococcosis or toxoplasmosis), which can result in diminished cognitive capacities and reduced ability to cope with life events.

The potential role of stress and depression as cofactors in mediating the development and course of the AIDS syndrome makes psychoneuroimmunology a promising area of scientific investigation. Hence the AIDS crisis has created a surge of scientific interest in psychoneuroimmunology for several reasons. First, AIDS is driving a new intensity of basic research on cellular and molecular functions, particularly of the immune and nervous systems. This has contributed to rapid research advances, revealing unexpected complexities in possible psychoneuroimmune linkages. Second, AIDS appears to have important psychological and behavioral components ("cofactors") that may be critical in understanding etiology and in the development of effective treatments. Third, AIDS has resisted our efforts to understand it in terms of conventional biomedical concepts. Like cancer, schizophrenia, and cardiovascular disease, where behavioral factors are critical to the development and course of these illnesses, the AIDS epidemic is pushing us toward a new biomedical paradigm that incorporates biological, psychological, and social factors in our understanding of the disease. This, in fact, is the more holistic orientation of psychoneuroimmunology.

The value of a psychoneuroimmunologic approach to research on AIDS has been recognized, especially as data accumulate documenting CNS, endocrine, ANS, and immune changes observed with states of depression and hopelessness that might influence the activation of, and the course of, AIDS. After transmission HIV can exist in a latent, non replicating form. Activation is related to a "tat" gene that is responsible for transacting transcriptional activation.[73,78] AIDS becomes a clinical problem when viral genes are activated and new virus particles are formed which then infect fresh T4 cells—one of HIV's primary targets.

Researchers have wondered whether stress could activate HIV from a latent to a rapidly replicating state.[1,76] It has been proposed that stress may be one of several possible activators of the "tat" gene and HIV. Psychological stress is thought to be involved in the activation of latent herpes simplex virus. A key question is, What activates viral genes? A widely held notion is that further challenges to the immune system by another infection are responsible. Examples of such agents include intestinal parasites, cytomegalovirus,

Epstein-Barr virus, and coexisting sexually transmitted diseases such as syphilis and gonorrhea. Other proposed cofactors include the use of steroids or antineoplastic agents, nutritional deficiency states, age, alcohol intake, ionizing radiation, and exposure to certain chemicals.[78-80]

It is likely that predisposition to HIV infection and the development of AIDS is multifactorial. The psychological status of an individual may function as a mediator through the immune system to activate latent virus or contribute to the infection taking hold. Therefore, the disease may also proceed more rapidly in a person whose immune system is already impaired by drugs or infection. Possibly, changes associated with endocrine and CNS activity, triggered by stressful life events and emotional reactions, could also impair the immune system or operate as a cofactor.

Certain host-susceptibility factors may also increase the risk of AIDS or be responsible for activating dormant virus. Some of these factors may explain why some people with active HIV infection deteriorate rapidly and die while others have a less virulent course. Recognizing that emotional states may have powerful influences on immune function and disease outcome, a number of questions arise. How are people affected when they learn of their seropositivity? Will knowledge of viral infection produce a psychological state that could set in motion biological changes that might activate the virus? Subjects with AIDS and at high risk for AIDS become fearful as well as depressed. In addition, they are subject to major losses that lead to intense grief and major alterations in their social environment and finally to feeling abandoned and uncertain. Thus it is not surprising that psychoneuroendocrinological factors relating to the progression of AIDS and AIDS-related illnesses have come under investigation.

This area of study underscores the necessity of replicating in other populations Kiecolt-Glasser's paradigm that psychosocial interventions can normalize alterations in some immune parameters in medical students.[81,82] It also indicates the importance of intense study of immune parameters in subjects at risk for particular illnesses to determine which variables are reversible, which predict progression to disease, and which are early manifestations of illness as compared to late secondary phenomenon of disease state.

In view of the viral etiology of AIDS, recent studies are of interest: the effects of medical school–associated stress on viral infection of lymphoid cells in vitro and reactivation of viral infection in vivo.[81-84] These studies reported increased Epstein-Barr virus transformability of B cells in vitro (in a mixed T- and B-cell preparation in which the T cells generally inhibit transformation) in response to medical school examinations, increased stress, and high loneliness ratings. Similar psychosocial responses were associated with increased titers of antibodies directed against several herpes viruses that the authors associate with reactivation of latent virus. These results, if confirmed (and if viral titers are truly a marker of reactivation), complement earlier clinical studies in humans that indicate stress may increase susceptibility to other viral illnesses such as mononucleosis and trenchmouth.

Solomon and Temoshok found that differences in disease outcome in AIDS patients apparently parallel the scientific literature findings on helplessness and hopelessness.[76] Patients dying more quickly of AIDS had a lower score on a control measure, suggesting that they tend to feel powerless in the face of overwhelming forces. Further, the unfavourable outcome group had less utilization of assistance for problem solving. These findings suggest the importance of counseling and psychotherapy not only for improving the patient's mood and quality of life but also in managing the biological consequences of the viral infection.

However, it should be underscored that AIDS is an extremely difficult illness to study because of the number of factors influencing its course and development and its profound effect on the immune system. These factors seriously impede the determination of whether immune alterations are caused by stress or disease progression. Additionally, it is difficult to determine which of these immune parameters are markers of illness and which are indicators of susceptibility and vulnerability. Even in subjects with fully developed cases of AIDS, it is not clear which immune alterations are intrinsic to the illness and which are phenomena secondary to diminished immune function and/or dysregulation. With respect to intervention, it is unclear at which stage the illness (i.e., progression from exposure to virus, asymptomatic viral infection, AIDS-related complex [ARC], or clinical AIDS syndrome) is most amenable to psychosocial interventions that might modulate immune function.

THE BIOLOGY OF HOPE AND POSITIVE EMOTIONS: IMPLICATIONS FOR TREATMENT

The past few decades have seen an increasing awareness that various emotions —rather than relating to a singular state of arousal—may be associated with different psychophysiological states. What is beginning to emerge is the belief that if negative emotions are associated with negative psychophysiological states (in terms of their consequences), then it may be reasonable to postulate that positive emotions may correlate with positive psychophysiological changes. Therefore, researchers now believe that different emotions exert different effects across the mind–brain interface. A considerable number of studies, including some already mentioned, have suggested the biological impact and often health-damaging consequences of emotional states including depression, despair, hopelessness, and helplessness.[1,4,14,53,63,84] Currently, however, little data, are available to support the potential health-enhancing effects of positive emotions and to formulate a biology of hope, although many anecdotes and clinical observations support the possibility of such effects. If life stress and negative emotional states can cause immune suppression and possibly increase vulnerability to illness, then conceivably positive states such as psychosocial support, positive emotions, hope, and humor might enhance immune function, potentiate recovery, and increase resistance to immunologically related illnesses.

Cousins vividly and dramatically suggested the healing effects of hope, humor, and a sense of mastery in chronicling the history of his own serious illness.[85,86] His publications remind us that positive emotions, as well as a message of hopefulness from an authoritative, benevolent, caring figure, whether doctor, a healer, or a family member, may not only create a sense of well-being in the patient but set in motion reparative biological processes. Expectant faith in ultimate recovery is further increased by the conviction that the patient shares with the healer and the community a set of assumptions about the cause of illness and the appropriate treatment. The therapeutic ritual may provide a plan of action for the patient, family, and community that gives them all a sense of purpose and mastery.

Clinicians and scientists have begun to examine improvements in clinical states associated with faith, hope, meditation, humor, and psychotherapy. Relief of pain and euphoria are other features of so-called healing practices that researchers suggest could result from endogenous endorphins. The therapeutic effects of healing practices have often been ascribed to a "placebo" effect. Interestingly, endorphins have been suggested as a possible biological mediator of such placebo effects. Benson suggested that the relaxation response from yoga, meditation, and prayer may have its healing source in an integrated hypothalamic response that results in a generalized decrease in sympathetic nervous system activity.[87] Several preliminary studies reported alterations of a variety of human immune parameters using behavioral interventions including hypnosis, suggestion, "imagery," relaxation procedures, and biofeedback.[88]

Unfortunately, these studies have methodological problems, and some have not been replicated. Even if it were demonstrated that healthy people can self-regulate aspects of their immune system, additional evidence would be necessary to demonstrate that such changes can prevent or cure illness. It is still not clear whether psychotherapeutic or behavioral interventions can directly enhance immune function and thereby influence the onset or course of diseases thought to be associated with abnormal immune function.

Other examples come from the literature on the clinical course of cancer. Some cancer patients survive much longer than expected; others die more quickly than predicted.[89,90] The long survivors have been noted by some to be less anxious and depressed and to show faith and inner confidence—they are often people who state from the onset that they will fight the disease. Persons who die sooner than expected have been described as seemingly helpless and full of despair. Some cancer patients who had utilized relaxation techniques and mental imagery were observed by Hall to show some evidence of attenuation of their cancer.[91]

Levy and Cohorts described a study that tested the predictive power of baseline psychological and behavioral measures to determine whether they accounted for any of the outcome variance in breast cancer patients as reflected by time to recurrence in patients treated with somatic treatments.[92] Patients' scores on mood and social support variables predicted the direction of NK activity three months after baseline treatment.

Kiecolt-Glaser and colleagues reported the enhancement of immunocompetence through relaxation techniques utilized by 45 geriatric patients.[81] In contrast to a social contact and control group, the group provided with the relaxation paradigm showed an increase in natural killer cell activity and a decrease in titers to herpes simplex virus. T-cell response to mitogen stimulation also increased. These investigators additionally reported immune enhancement via relaxation techniques in medical student subjects. These research studies suggest that psychological interventions may modify the effects of life stress and negative emotions on immune function.

CONCLUSION

The studies mentioned in the preceding section raise the question of whether certain psychosocial factors and emotional states—including happiness, security, humor, a sense of control, a fighting spirit, psychological hardiness, determination, social support, and other positive emotions—are associated with biological changes that can induce good health, remission from serious illness, or enhanced response to treatment. A definitive answer requires psychobiological research on the effects of behavioral and psychosocial interventions on specific aspects of immune function and overall physical health. Currently, AIDS research needs a biopsychosocial rather than a biomedical model, and this perspective must be maintained even when studies emphasize elucidating pathophysiological mechanisms and search for vaccines and new chemotherapies for treating the disease. Medical research has a history of delaying investigatory studies in what appears to be soft research or humanistic concerns and instead embarks on the enticing search for the magic bullet.

These remarks are not meant to imply that the research community should decrease the study of the development and use of antiviral drugs or vaccines for AIDS. Rather, if our research is to be guided by an integrative model, then investigations of pharmacologic agents would automatically incorporate into the research design studies of psychosocial and CNS factors that might influence the response to these drugs.

In spite of the difficulty in relinquishing a biomedical model, it is hoped that AIDS-related research will facilitate a more integrated biopsychosocial systems model to replace the archaic dualistic mind-body model that still dominates our concept of disease. It is also hoped that health professionals will recognize (1) that AIDS and AIDS-related issues must become part of the mainstream of our clinical, research, and educational activities and not be treated as a curiosity to be segregated to a small number of interested people and (2) that the integrative biopsychosocial model must be updated and used by health professionals.

One extremely important and serendipitous outcome of AIDS research has been biological data suggesting specific mechanisms that mediate mind-body interactions. The work of Pert and colleagues is an example.[93] Pert showed that the T4 immunocyte surface receptor that binds and human immunodeficiency virus is common to specific areas of the brain. The anatomical pattern of the brain receptors is similar to that for certain neuropeptide transmitter systems thought to play a central role in complex functions such as emotion. Pert's group has identified an octapeptide ("peptide T") from the HIV envelope-protein sequence that inhibits virus binding and is found in the sequence of an endogenous hormone and, likely, neuropeptide VIP (vasoactive intestinal peptide).

Beyond providing clues about direct infection of the brain by HIV, this work may implicate biopsychosocial systems research. Here we have a glimpse of a possible process that ties together cell surface recognition, neuropeptides, probable genetic transformation, a disease with gross neuropsychiatric effects, and interactions between the immune and nervous systems.

We are in great need of new conceptual approaches. Many of the research studies and methods described in this chapter may suggest a new way of thinking about disease, treatment, and prevention at the whole organism level. Additionally, psychoimmunologic studies may provide evidence of both the biological and psychological impact of psychosocial interventions. Conceivably we may be able to develop and tailor specific perceptual, cognitive, and behavioral interventions for specific patient populations as adjunct therapies to enhance other therapeutic modalities. We may find, in fact, that the combination of psychosocial and pharmacologic treatments for disease increases therapeutic benefits for the patient.

Indeed, this time may be very propitious for health care professionals to examine more carefully and consider the theoretical justification and empirical evidence for the role of psychosocial and psychologically meaningful medical interventions in the armamentarium against major physical disorders that are incapacitating, painful, deforming, and currently not entirely preventable or curable. If some of these techniques (e.g., hypnosis, imagery, meditation, biofeedback) are useful in the treatment of physical disorders, then these therapeutic strategies must be conceptualized and incorporated into health care programs. Similarly, research must be designed and implemented to study their mechanism of action and test their effectiveness.

Health care professionals who remain at least dimly aware that everything they do or say to a patient conveys a major or minor, positive or negative, helpful or harmful, psychological impact are likely to be more effective health care providers. If this dim awareness can be heightened to a set of conscious, organized, definable principles, the whole health care system may be able to deliver more effective, comprehensive, and compassionate health care.

REFERENCES

1. Solomon G: The emerging field of psychoneuroimmunology. Advances, Institutes for the Advancement of Health 2(1):6–19, 1985.
2. Cunningham AJ: "Gestalt immunology": A less reductionist approach to the subject. In: Bell GI, Perelson AS, Pimbley GH (eds) Theoretical Immunology. New York: Marcel Dekker, 1978.
3. Cunningham AJ: Some similarities in the way the immune system and nervous system work. In: The Immune System, Vol. 1. Switzerland: Basel-Karger, 1981.
4. Regan B: Psychoneuroimmunology: The birth of a new field. Investigations—A Bulletin of the Institute of Noetic Sciences 1(2), 1983.
5. Ishigami T: The influence of psychic acts on the progress of pulmonary tuberculosis. Am Rev Tuberc 2:470–484, 1918–1919.
6. Jensen M, Rasmussen A: Stress and susceptibility to viral infection. Immunol 90(1):17–20, 1963.
7. Johnsson T, Lavender J, Hulton E, Rasmussen A. The influence of avoidance learning stress on resistance to coxsackie B virus in mice. J Immunol 91:569–579, 1963.
8. Marsh JT, Lavender JF, Shueh-Shen C, Rasmussen AF: Poliomyelitis in monkeys: Decreased susceptibility after avoidance stress. Science 140(3574):1414–1415, 1968.
9. Imboden JB, Canter A, Cluff LE: Convalescence from influenza. Arch Intern Med 108:393–399, 1961.
10. Meyer RJ, Haggerty RV: Streptococcal infections in families. Pediatrics 30(4):539–549, 1962.
11. Solomon G, Moos R: The relationship of personality to the presence of rheumatoid factor in asymptomatic relatives in patients with rheymatoid arthritis. Psychosom Med 27:350–360, 1965.
12. Dougherty TF, Frank JA: The qualitative and quantitative responses of blood lymphocytes to stress stimuli. J Lab Clin Med 42(4):530–537, 1953.
13. Gisler RH, Schenkel-Hulliger L: Hormonal regulation of the immune response: Influence of pituitary and adrenal activity on immune responsiveness in vitro. Cell Immunol 2:646–657, 1971.
14. Besedovsky J. Sorkin E, Felex D, Haas H: Hypothalamic changes during the immune response. Eur J Immunol 7(5):323–325, 1977.
15. Jankovic BD, Isakovic K: Neuroendocrine correlates of immune response. Int Arch All App Immunol 45:369–372, 1973.
16. Filip G, Szentivany I, Moss B: Anaphylaxis and the nervous system, Acta Med Acad Sci, TOM III FASI 2:103, 1952.
17. Mihailovic L, Jankovic B: Effects of intraventricularly injected anti-n caudatus antibody on the electrical activity of the cat brain. Nature 192(4803)665–666, 1961.
18. Korneva E, Khai L: The effect of the destruction of areas within the hypothalamic region on the process of immunogenesis. Sechenov Physiolog J USSR XLIX (1), 1963.
19. Lupurello T, Stein M, Paris CD: Effect of hypothalamic lesions on rat anaphylaxis. Am J Physiol 207:911–914, 1964.
20. Jankovic BC, Rakic E, Vaskov R, Horrat I. Effect of intraventricular injection of antibrain antibody on defensive conditional reflexes. Nature 218(5138):270–271, 1968.
21. Besedovsky HO, del Rey A, Sorkin E, DaPrada M, Keller HH. Immunoregulation mediated by the sympathetic nervous system. Cell Immunol 48:346–355, 1979.
22. Besedovsky H, Sorkin E: Network of immuno-neuroendocrine interactions. Clin Exp Immunol 27:1–12, 1977.
23. Bartrop RW, Lazarus L, Luckhurst E, Kiloh LG, Penny R: Depressed lymphocyte function after bereavement. Lancet 1:834–836, 1977.
24. Kasl S, Evans A, Niederman JC: Psychosocial risk factors with development of infectious mononucleosis. Psychosom Med 41(6):445–466, 1979.
25. Dameshek W: The white blood cells in dementia preocox and dementia parolytica. Arch Neurol Psychi 24:855, 1930.
26. Fessel WJ. Hiratu-Hiki M: Abnormal leukocytes in schizophrenia. Arch Gen Psychi 9:601–613, 1963.
27. Heath R, Krupp IM, Byers LW, Liljekust JI: Schizophrenia as an immunologic disorder. Arch Gen Psychi 16:24–33, 1967.

28. Solomon G, Moos R, Fessel WJ, Morgan EC: Globulins and behavior in schizophrenia. Intern J Neuropsych 2:20–26, 1966.
29. Vartanian ME, Kolyaskma DV, Lozovsky D, Biabaeva GS, Ignatov S: Aspects of humoral and cellular immunity in schizphrenia. In: Gergsam D, Goldstein AL (eds) Neurochemical and Immunologic Components of Schizophrenia. New York: A.R. Liss, pp 339–364, 1973.
30. Solomon GF, Levine S, Kraft KJ: Early experience and immunity. Nature 220(5169):821–822, 1968.
31. Solomon GF: Stress and antibody response in rats. Arch All App Immunol 35:97–104, 1969.
32. Dolin AO, Krylor VR, Luklianeko V, Flerov B: New experimental data on the conditioned reflex reproduction and suppression of immune and allergic reactions. ZH Vyssh Nervn Deyatel 10(6):832–841, 1960.
33. Ader R, Cohen N: Behaviorally conditioned immunosuppression. Psychosom Med 37:4:333–340, 1975.
34. Ader R (ed): Psychoneuroimmunology. New York: Academic Press, 1981.
35. Locke SE, Hornig-Rohan M: Mind and Immunity: Behavioral Immunology. An annotated bibliography 1976–82. New York: Institute for the Advancement of Health, 1983.
36. Locke S, Ader R, Besedovsky H, Hall N, Solomon G, Strom T: Foundations of Psychoneuroimmunology. New York: Aldine, 1985.
37. Spector NH, Korneva EA: Neurophysiology, immunophysiology and neuroimmunomodualation. In: Ader R (ed) Psychoneuroimmunology. New York: Academic Press, pp 449–473, 1981.
38. Spector NH: The central state of the hypothalamus in health and disease: Old and new concepts. In: Morgane PJ, Panskepp J (eds) Handbook of the Hypothalamus, Vol. 2. New York: Marcel Dekker, pp 453–517, 1980.
39. Stein M, Schleifer S, Keller S: Hypothalamic influence on immune responses. In: Ader R (ed) Psychoneuroimmunology. New York: Academic Press, pp 429–448, 1981.
40. Roszman T, Cross R, Brooks W. Markesberry, W: Hypothalamic-immune interaction. Immunology 45(4):737–742, 1982.
41. Gorman J, Locke S: Neural, endocrine and immune interactions. In: Kaplan H, Sydock B, (eds) Comprehensive Textbook of Psychiatry V. Baltimore: Williams & Wilkins, 1987.
42. Besedovsky H, del Rey A, Sorkin E, Dinarello CA: Immunoregulatory feedback between interleukin-1 and gluccorticoid hormones. Science 344(4764):652–654, 1986.
43. Ader R: A historical account of conditioned immunobiologic responses. In: Psychoneuroimmunology, New York: Academic Press, pp 321–352, 1981.
44. Rogers MP, Reich P, Strom TB, Carpenter CE: Behaviorally conditioned immunosuppression: Replication of a recent study. Psychosom Med 38:447–452, 1976.
45. Wayner EA, Flannery GR, Singer G: The effects of taste aversion conditioning on the primary antibody response to sheep red blood cells and Brucella abortus in the albino rat. Physiological Behavior 21:995–1000, 1978.
46. Bovbjerg D, Ader R, Cohen N: Behaviorally conditioned supression of a graft-versus-host response. Pro Nat Acad Sci USA 79:583–585, 1982.
47. Solvason HB, Ghanta V, Hiramoto R, Spector NH: Natural killer cell activity augmented by classical Pavlovian conditioning. First International Workshop on Neuroimmunology, 1984.
48. Ader R, Cohen N: Behaviorally conditioned immunosuppression and murine systemic lupus erthematosus. Science 215:1534–1536, 1982.
49. Gorczynski R: Analysis of lymphocytes in and host environment of mice showing conditioned immunosuppression to cyclo phosphamide. Brain Behav Immun 1:21–35, 1987.
50. Spector NH: Old and new strategies in the conditioning of immune responses. Ann NY Acad Sci 62:74, 1987.
51. Selye H: The Stress of Life. New York: McGraw-Hill, 1976.
52. Kaufman I, Rosenbaum LA: The reaction to separation in infant monkeys. Psychosom Med 29:648–675, 1975.
53. Engel GL: Sudden and rapid death during psychological stress: Folklore or folkwisdom. Ann Intern Med 74(5):771–778, 1971.
54. DeSilva R. Central nervous system risk factors for sudden cardiac death. In: Greenberg HM, Dwyer EM (eds) Sudden Cardiac Death. New York: New York Academy of Science, 382:143–161, 1982.

55. Lown B, Psychophysiologic factors in sudden cardiac death. Am J Psychi 137(11):1325–1335, 1980.
56. Binik Y. Sudden death in the laboratory rat. Psychosom Med 39:82–93, 1977.
57. Corley KC: Cardiac responses associated with "yoked chair" shock avoidance in Squirrel Monkeys. Psychophysiology 12(4):439–444, 1975.
58. Corley KC: Myocardial degeneration and cardiac arrest in Squirrel Monkeys. Psychophysiology 3:322–328, 1977.
59. Richter CP: On the phenomena of sudden death in animals and man. Psychosom Med 19:101–108, 1957.
60. Riley V, Fitzmaurice M, Spackman DH: Psychoneuroimmunologic factors in neoplasia. In: Ader R (ed) Psychoneuroimmunology. New York: Academic Press, pp 31–102, 1981.
61. Seligman M: Helplessness. San Francisco: W.H. Freeman, 1976.
62. Laudenslanger ML, Ryan SM, Drugan RC, Hyson RL, Maier SF: Coping and immunosuppression: Inescapable but not escapable shock suppresses lymphocyte proliferation. Science 221:568–70, 1983.
63. Stein M: A biopsychosocial approach to immune function and medical disorders. Psychia Clin NA 4(2):203–221, 1981.
64. Post R: Potential of neuroscience research. In Pincus AA, Purdiev A., The Integration of Neuroscience and Psychiatry, Chapter 2. Washington DC: APA Press, 1985.
65. Anisman H: Vulnerability to depression: Contribution of stress. In: Post R, Bullough JC (eds) Neurobiology of Mood Disorders. Baltimore: Williams & Wilkins, 1986.
66. Schleifer SJ, Keller SE, Stein N: Stress effects of immunity. Psychiatric J U Ottawa 10(3):125–131, 1985.
67. Irwin M, Daniels M, Bloom ET, Smith JC, Weiner HT: Life events, depression symptoms and immune function. Am J Psychia 144(4):437–441, 1987.
68. Pert C, Ruff M, Weber R, Herkenham M: Neuropeptides and their receptors: A psychosomatic network. J Immuno 135(2):820S–826S, 1985.
69. Ruff MR, Pert CE: Small cell carcinoma of the lung: Macrophage specific antigens suggest hemopoietic stem cell origin. Science 225:1034–1086, 1984.
70. Bullock K: Neuroanatomy of lymphoid tissue. In: Guillemin R, Cohn M, Melnechuk T (eds) Neural Modulation of Immunity. New York: Raven Press, pp 111–141, 1985.
71. Renoux G, Biziere K: Brain neocortex lateralized control of immune regulation. Integrative Psychiatry 4(1):32–36, 1986.
72. Besedovsky J, Sorkin B: Immunologic-neuroendocrine circuits. In: Adler R (ed) Psychoneuroimmunology. New York: Academic Press, pp 545–574, 1981.
73. Besedovsky J, del Rey A, Sorkin E, DaPrada M, Burri R, Honegger C: The immune response evokes changes in brain noradrenergic neurons. Science 221:564–566, 1983.
74. Smith EM, Meyer WJ, Blalock JE: Virus-induced cortico sterone in hypophysectomized mice: A possible lymphoid adrenal axis. Science 218:1311–1312, 1982.
75. Hall NR, McGillis J, Spangelo B, Goldstein AL: Evidence that thymosin and other biologic response modifiers can function as neuroactive immunotransmitters. J Immunol 135(3):806S–811S, 1985.
76. Solomon G, Temoshok L: A psychoneuroimmunologic perspective on AIDS research. J App Soc Psychol 17(3):286–308, 1987.
77. Folks T, Posell DM, Lightfoote MM, Benn S, Martin HA, Fauci AS: Induction of HTLV/LAV from a non-virus producing T-cell line. Science 231:600–602, 1986.
78. Sodorski JG, Rosen CA, Haseltine WR: Transacting, transcription of the long terminal report of human T-lymphocyte viruses in infected cells. Science 225:381, 1984.
79. Curran JW, et al: The epidemiology of AIDS: Current status and future prospects. Science, 605–617, 1985.
80. Fauci AS, Macher AM, Longo DI: Acquired immunodeficiency syndrome: Epidemiologic, clinical, immunologic and therapeutic considerations. Ann Int Med 100:92–106, 1983.
81. Kiecolt-Glaser J, Glaser R, Williger D. Stout J, Messick G, Shappard S, Ricker D, Romisher S, Brinev W, Bonnell G, Donnerberg R: Psychosocial enhancement of immunocompetence in a geriatric population. Health Psychology 4(1):25–41, 1985.
82. Kiecolt-Glaser J, Glaser R: Psychosocial moderators of immune function. Ann Behav Med 9:16–20, 1987.
83. Glaser R, Kiecolt-Glaser J, Speicher CE, Holliday JE: Stress, loneliness and changes in herpes virus latency. J Behav Med 8:249–260, 1985.

84. Glaser R, Rice J. Sheridan J, Fertil R, Stout J, Speicher C, Pinsky D, Kutur M, Post A, Beck M, Kiecolt-Glaser J: Stress-related immune suppression: Health implications. Brain Behav Immun 1:7–20, 1987.
85. Cousins N: Anatomy of an Illness. New York: W.W. Norton, 1979.
86. Consins N: The Healing Heart. New York: W.W. Norton, 1983.
87. Benson H: The relaxation response and norepinephrine. Integrative Psychiatry 1:15–18, 1983.
88. Locke S, Gorman J: Behavior and immunity. In: Kaplan H, Sadock B (eds) Comprehensive Textbook of Psychiatry, V. Baltimore: Williams & Wilkins, 1987.
89. Blumberg EM, Nest PM, Ellis FN: A possible relationship between psychological factors and human cancer. Psychosom Med 16:276, 1954.
90. Borysenko J: Behavioral and physiological factors in the development and management of cancer. Gen Hosp Psychiat 4:69–74, 1982.
91. Hall H: Imagery and cancer. In Sheikh AA (ed) Imagination and Healing. Farmingdale, NY: Baywood, 1984.
92. Levy S, Herberman R, Lippman M, d'Angelo J: Correlation of stress factors with sustained depression of natural killer cell activity and predicted prognosis on patients with breast cancer. J Clin Oncol 5(3):348–353, 1987.
93. Pert C: Neuropeptides: The emotions and body mind. Noetic Sciences Review 2:12–18, 1987.

3. ANESTHETIC MANAGEMENT OF AIDS PATIENTS

ERNEST R. GREENE, JR. AND THOMAS JANISSE

All we know is still infinitely less than all that still remains unknown.
WILLIAM HARVEY, DE MOTU CORDES ET SANGUINIS, 1628

As the human immunodeficiency virus (HIV) epidemic continues to make inroads into the general public, anesthesiologists face an ever-increasing number of infected persons. Some have full-blown AIDS, some are known to be HIV-positive, but most by far are undiagnosed.

How can these unfortunates best be handled? What is the proper role of regional anesthesia in their care? Despite the enormous quantity of information concerning HIV and its associated diseases, remarkably little has been written on this topic.[1-4] Controlled studies concerning possible advantages of regional versus general anesthesia have not been done. Useful published guidelines based on either experience or thoughtful consideration are scarce. Basic information concerning the frequency of use of regional versus general anesthesia by practitioners is simply unavailable.

Would the availability of such information lead to better patient care? Doubtless it would. An interchange of information on this incompletely understood set of diseases could only serve to benefit the patients thus afflicted. This chapter may help to stimulate the process by which the anesthesia community learns to deal effectively with this group of patients and the diseases they face.

OVERVIEW

The state of health of patients infected by HIV varies widely. At the one extreme, some of those suffering from full-blown AIDS are critically ill and subject to severe decompensation from even a mild anesthetic insult. At the other, many of those who, despite infection, still have a largely intact immune system are in robust good health without the least outward sign of disease.

The question exists whether some particular anesthetic might serve as a cofactor of AIDS. That is, whether that agent might cause a reactivation of latent HIV lodged within a T lymphocyte or other host cell. Cofactors do exist, but anesthetic agents are not thought to be included among their number. Medicolegally, one can make a case that certain blocks might be ill-advised, if not actually harmful, but this is another matter and will be considered later. With these reservations, there may be no compelling medical reasons to treat the healthy, infected patient differently from the healthy, uninfected one. Furthermore, each day hundreds or thousands of persons who are infected with undetected HIV are routinely anesthetized, with no attention given to this underlying condition. No retrospective study has been done to suggest that their disease processes were affected by these anesthetics. Indeed, such a study would be difficult to do and difficult to interpret, particularly in light of the long incubation period of AIDS.

What this chapter addresses is largely sick patients with severe immunosuppression who need anesthesia for any condition, whether it be related to their underlying infection or not. Consideration is also given to those patients with early HIV infection in whom anesthetic management may differ based on their initial clinical presentation. For all patients the anesthesiologist needs to focus on preexisting conditions via a careful preanesthetic assessment. This approach, concentrating on a good history and physical examination, remains the most rational way to decide whether regional or general anesthesia is best for a particular patient.

Anesthetic care extends beyond the confines of the operative suite. Today, anesthesiologists are more involved with extended postoperative pain relief than they were formerly. Patients with AIDS often have a preexisting baseline of pain and may benefit expecially from this newer service.

Regional analgesia for patients with AIDS who have a chronic pain syndrome will be addressed in chapter 6. The general principles discussed later concerning matters such as the control of infection apply as well for blocks performed for chronic pain as for surgical anesthesia.

The potential exists for the transmission of an HIV infection to a member of the hospital staff or to another patient. Transmission rarely happens, but when it does it is a catastrophe to those affected. Of particular importance, to help protect the staff and to ensure strict adherence to universal precautions, the anesthesiologist has a responsibility to educate other operating room and pain clinic personnel about the possible presentation of a person with HIV infection. Helpful guidelines will be presented to minimize the chances of inadvertant HIV transmission.

Table 3-1. Initial clinical presentations of HIV infection

Gastrointestinal	Nausea/vomiting
	Abdominal pain
	Diarrhea
General	Weight loss
	Malaise
	Edema
	Sepsis
Neurologic	Headache
	Seizure
	Syncope
	Truncal rash
	Limb weakness
	Myalgia
Orofacial	Palate/tongue lesions
	Parotid swelling
	7th nerve palsy
	Cervical adenitis
Psychiatric	Behavioral change
	Major depression
	Dementia
Pulmonary	Cough
	Fever
	Chest pain
Renal	Azotemia
Trauma	Accidental fall
	Fracture

GENERAL ANESTHETIC MANAGEMENT

Anesthesiologists should be particularly aware of the initial clinical presentations of people with HIV infection, as listed in table 3-1, because these may not be immediately considered as HIV infection. People infected with HIV may have multisystem involvement and dysfunction. The anesthesiologist, when developing the anesthetic plan—whether for regional or general anesthesia, must consider the many problems present in these people or that may occur suddenly and unexpectedly, even in those thought to be free of HIV infection. Table 3-2 lists the possible clinical problems or concerns in the order that an anesthesiologist may encounter them. The following discussion expands selected points in this table.

Patients with AIDS often come to surgery in very bad condition.

They may have severe respiratory problems,[5,6] at times associated with hypoxia, due to pulmonary diseases such as Pneumocystis carinii pneumonia,[7-9] pulmonary alveolar proteinosis,[10] pulmonary Kaposi's sarcoma,[11,12] cytomegalovirus pneumonitis,[13] pulmonary cryptococcosis,[14] lymphocytic interstitial pneumonia,[15] and histoplasmosis.[16] Once intubated and mechanically ventilated, many of these patients are very difficult to wean from respiratory support. It is helpful for the anesthesiologist to speak to the

Table 3–2. Chronologic list of clinical HIV associations

PREOPERATIVE VISIT

Anemia	Azidothymidine (AZT) effect
Ataxia, paresis	Vacuolar myelopathy
Azotemia	Nephropathy
Behavior (high risk)	HIV infection
Cough	Bronchitis or pneumonitis from opportunistic infection
Dysesthesias/paresthesias (distal)	Predominantly sensory neuropathy (PSN); herpes zoster (HZ)
Fatigue	Anemia; electrolyte imbalance from vomiting or diarrhea
Fever, headache	Aseptic meningitis
Mentation (altered)	HIV encephalopathy; increased intracranial pressure from a mass
Plaques (white, tongue)	Oral hairy leukoplakia
Papules (red, palate)	Kaposi's sarcoma
Radiculopathy	Herpes zoster
Syncope, orthostatic hypotension	Autonomic neuropathy; dehydration
Weakness (motor)	Guillain-Barré syndrome (GBS)

RESUSCITATION

Intubation, catheters	Fluid exposure; induce infection
Traumatic wounds	Fluid exposure

PREINDUCTION

Catheters	Fluid exposure; induce infection
Peridural access	Thrombocytopenia, coagulation abnormalites, progressive neurologic disease; immune compromise, induce bacterial infection; assess peripheral nervous system

INDUCTION

Analgesics	May suppress immune function; tolerance from intravenous drug abuse
Hypnosedatives or inhalation agents	Exacerbate encephalopathy; oversensitivity from CNS disease
Oxygen	Compensate for V/Q mismatch (opportunistic infection)
Succinylcholine	Hyperkalemia from neuromuscular disease or vacuolar myelopathy
Enflurane	Seizure
Nitrous oxide	Leukopenia
Nondepolarizing muscle relaxants	Aberrant neuromuscular function (NM junction spared)
Cardiac arrest	Autonomic neuropathy

INTRAOPERATIVE

Oxygen	Oxygen desaturation from pulmonary disease; compromised CNS function; anemia
Analgesics	Narcotics vs. local anesthetics
Arrhythmias	Antiviral drug interaction or side effects; cocaine abuse
Ventricular failure	Wall motion or valve abnormalities; pericardial effusion; cardiomyopathy
Aerosolized blood	Orthopedic or cardiothoracic surgery
Liver metabolism	Alcohol abuse, antifungal agents

EMERGENCE

Extubation	Fluid exposure; prolonged ventilation

POSTOPERATIVE

Analgesics	Opiates vs. local anesthetic; consider best opiate route
Assessment	Neurologic alterations (CNS/PNS)

surgeon, to the primary care physician, to the patient, and to his or her family concerning this matter. In some cases those involved with the patient's primary care would like to avoid the complications of intubation and ventilation, and so the opportunity to proceed with a regional anesthetic may be relatively attractive. Such patients should receive the minimal amount of sedative to avoid respiratory depression and the level of their spinal or epidural block, should one be given, ought to be no higher than needed. Supplemental oxygen should be used, and a pulse oximeter is advisable. Preoperative blood gases are important, and an arterial line may be helpful in safely getting intraoperative arterial blood samples with a minimum number of needle sticks. All these patients should have a preoperative chest x-ray.

Patients with AIDS or even ARC are often grossly dehydrated, malnourished, and electrolytically imbalanced due to vomiting, diarrhea, and anorexia. The signs of dehydration, such as orthostatic hypotension, decreased skin turgor, and dry tongue, should be sought in all sick AIDS patients. These dehydrated patients are often hemodynamically only borderline stable or even frankly unstable and unable to tolerate a general anesthetic, a spinal, or an epidural. Even a major peripheral nerve block such as of the axillary plexus can be dangerous owing to the possibility of a complication such as an intravascular injection. Optimally, the surgeon should proceed with a purely local technique if possible. Otherwise, the patient should be carefully monitored with a central line and often with an arterial line as well. Cautious fluid repletion with the fluid of choice should be done before the induction of anesthesia or the institution of a major block.

Cardiomyopathies can occur in patients with AIDS,[17,18] thus necessitating extreme care with cardiac-depressant drugs and favoring the use of extensive invasive monitoring, perhaps including a pulmonary artery catheter. Such patients, depending on the site of their surgery, may benefit from a careful regional technique. However, they may poorly tolerate the magnitude of decreased blood pressure that often accompanies a spinal or an epidural, even one restricted to the lower extremities.

Medicolegally, as well as medically, it is prudent to document preoperatively whether the patient has an altered mental status or a neurological abnormality, common disorders in AIDS patients. Because opportunistic brain infections or intracranial tumors, with their mass effect, may lead to intracranial hypertension during anesthesia, appropriate techniques and drugs must be used. Seizures due to AIDS-related brain lesions are common, so enflurane should be used with particular caution. Paresis due to AIDS is a problem that may be seen. In such patients succinylcholine chloride may cause dangerous hyperkalemia and should therefore be avoided.

As discussed in chapter 1, the entire neuromuscular system except the neuromuscular junction seems vulnerable to HIV infection. Thus drug-receptor or drug-drug interactions may be normal at the neuromuscular junction, while the peripheral nerve and the muscle itself may function abnormally. The only safe approach is to assess muscle function grossly by physical examination and to test neuromuscular function with a peripheral nerve stimulator. A small dose of a short-acting, nondepolarizing muscle relaxant should be administered and its effect evaluated clinically and with a peripheral nerve stimulator. Since the person with polymyositis may have enough muscle injury to significantly elevate the serum creatinine kinase, hyperkalemia could be of concern in those with severe involvement, in which case succinylcholine should be avoided.

Since HIV is neurotropic, both centrally and peripherally, the range of neurological problems is broad. These include dysautonomia associated with orthostatic hypotension,[19] as discussed in chapter 1, dorsal root ganglioneuronitis yielding an ataxic neuropathy,[20] progressive inflammatory polyradiculopathy causing a severe cauda equina syndrome with eventual paraplegia,[21] meningitis caused directly by HIV,[22] and chronic inflammatory demyelinating polyneuropathy.[23]

An accidental fall may be the first clinical sign of HIV infection. Cheung and Weg reviewed accidental falls in hospitalized patients, aged 18 to 55, over a six-month period. Of the 29 patients found, 45% were IV drug abusers; the accidental fall was the first clinical manifestation of AIDS in 31%.[24]

Postoperatively, patients with AIDS have a high mortality rate. One study showed an astonishingly high mortality rate of 48% for elective surgery and 57% for emergency surgery.[25] The cause of death was usually progression of an opportunistic infection or a malignancy. Whether the stress of surgery and anesthesia might have led to an exacerbation of the underlying HIV infection in these patients is unknown. However, the impression that surgery may tip a seropositive patient into AIDS has been suggested in at least one case report.[26] To date, there is still no firm evidence that this is the case, although anesthetics have several unfavorable effects on the immune system.[27,28] A prolonged exposure to nitrous oxide results in leukopenia. Many anesthetics in conjunction with such factors as operative stress, blood transfusion, and hypotension may contribute to depressed T-cell function.[29,30]

Patients with AIDS should benefit from the improvements in postoperative pain care that are becoming available. For example, the use of patient-controlled analgesia (PCA) pumps is rapidly expanding. Aside from the excellent pain relief they provide owing to their manipulation by the patients themselves, these pumps provide an element of welcome control to those who often feel they retain little or none over their own lives.

To summarize the basic anesthetic management of patients with AIDS, many of whom may be quite ill, the following guidelines generally hold:

1. AIDS is a collection of diseases resulting from severe immune suppression. Neither regional nor general anesthesia is intrinsically better for all these patients due to the wide range of pathology that may be encountered.
2. The underlying condition of the patient dictates the anesthetic course. Thus

one avoids giving succinylcholine chloride to a paralyzed patient with AIDS as one would avoid it in one without AIDS.

3. No study has shown anesthesia to cause an exacerbation of a latent HIV infection.

4. One can expect general anesthetics to have roughly the equivalent effects on AIDS patients as on equally ill non-AIDS patients. More debilitated patients may be expected to require less of most drugs for an equivalent effect.

5. Infections, particularly of the central nervous system and the epidural space, are potentially severe problems in some patients with AIDS due to pre-existing systemic infections as well as to a depressed immune system. Scrupulous attention to sterile technique must be paid.

6. Because many patients with AIDS have or will develop neurological problems, it is prudent to discuss this particular issue with them before performing regional anesthesia.

7. Patients with AIDS may benefit considerably from careful postoperative pain management. PCA pumps may be especially well-received by this group.

The anesthetic management of patients with AIDS is complex and multifaceted. Good judgment in light of incomplete information on this issue demands that carefully informed consent be obtained before going on with a block. Eventually, the ratio of risks to benefits should become more clear. Other questions such as the effect of anesthetics on latent HIV infections await a definitive answer as well.

REGIONAL ANESTHETIC MANAGEMENT

The decision to give a regional or general anesthetic to a patient with HIV infection depends on many factors, primarily, the contraindications to regional anesthesia, and secondarily, the stage of HIV infection and its attendant pathophysiology. Both are considered together since they are interwoven; in general, the more evolved the HIV infection, the greater are the pathophysiologic changes and the greater the risk. A patient with AIDS for whom such blocks are considered should be warned of the increased risks associated with these procedures.

The following discussion covers three contraindications to a spinal or epidural regional anesthetic and how they relate to the person with HIV infection: systemic or local infection, progressive neurologic disease, and coagulation disorder.

Infection

All persons with AIDS have a severely deranged immune system and are considerably more apt than normal patients to acquire an infection from invasive procedures. Many, of course, actually come to surgery with an active

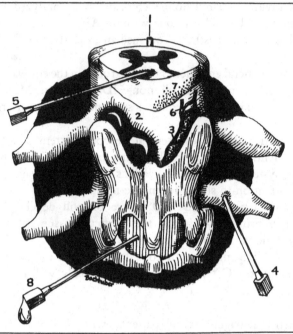

Figure 3–1. Routine potential peridural complications. **(1)** Anterior spinal artery occlusion. **(2)** Epidural hematoma. **(3)** Epidural abscess. **(4)** Spinal nerve root injury. **(5)** Spinal cord injury. **(6)** Intravascular injection of local anesthetic. **(7)** Infectious contamination of spinal fluid. **(8)** Dural puncture with headache or unplanned subarachnoid drug effect.

infection, and for some this infection is systemic in nature. The risk of performing a spinal or epidural anesthetic may be considerable, particularly on this latter group. Patients with signs or symptoms of bacteremia, fungemia, or some other type of blood-borne opportunistic organism should not receive either of these major blocks.

Likewise, local infection at the proposed site of needle puncture contraindicates this procedure. See figure 3–1. The earlier question of CNS involvement in HIV infection is now moot, replaced with the knowledge that the CNS, if not primarily infected, is so shortly thereafter. Thus the worry about seeding a sterile CSF with human immunodeficiency virus present in the blood or soft tissue during a dural or epidural puncture is of far less concern.

Any person presenting with a headache and HIV infection must be evaluated for aseptic meningitis and, if so diagnosed, must begin treatment before any anesthetic is delivered. A general anesthetic would be indicated to avoid the possibility of a superimposed bacterial meningitis. Meningitis and encephalitis can also result from the use of a spinal or epidural anesthetic in an AIDS patient having a systemic infection. Because of the impaired immune status of these patients, such an infection once established may be more difficult to treat than one in a normal patient.

One serious outcome could be an epidural abscess characterized by fever and back pain (either generalized or localized) and often by nuchal rigidity. This abscess could result from a local infection at the puncture site. However, Baker and colleagues looked at 39 serial cases of an epidural abscess and found only one related to an epidural block; all others were associated with endogenous infection.[31] In another study of 49 patients with an epidural abscess, Hancock found the most common infecting organism to be *Staphylococcus aureus*.[32]

The AIDS patient with severe immunocompromise has a higher risk of an epidural abscess because of leukopenia and a blunted inflammatory response. In the normal patient leukocytosis is generally seen, but this sign might be absent in some patients with AIDS. Treacy and co-workers[33] found leukopenia to be common in patients with HIV infection, with the degree of infection correlated with the severity of the disease. They found 23% of 925 HIV-positive patients leukopenic, with 20% granulocytopenic. Eighty-eight percent of AIDS patients were leukopenic at presentation. A left shift in the granulocytic series was common and believed to be a reflection of the clinical condition of the patient. Zon and Groopman[34] found both anemia and granulocytopenia in the majority of AIDS patients and suggested it resulted from hematopoietic suppressor substances and the effect of antibodies directed specifically against cells in the bone marrow. Treatment of an epidural abscess is urgent laminectomy to decompress the spinal cord and the use of antibiotics. Paraplegia is likely unless prompt action is taken.

A person with HIV infection but without leukopenia, fever, or other symptoms or signs of a systemic infection may have no increased risk of CNS or epidural infection from a spinal or epidural anesthetic. On the other hand, a person with AIDS with severe immunocompromise, systemic infection, and a low granulocyte count may be at great risk, but this risk may be less than that from a general anesthetic and prolonged ventilation in a patient with severe pulmonary infection. After choosing a regional anesthetic, emphasis must be on a scrupulously sterile technique and close follow-up.

Neurologic disease

Progressive neurologic disease contraindicates a spinal or epidural anesthetic because of possible disease exacerbation by local anesthetic effect on neurons or the process of signal conduction, including axonal conduction and synaptic neurotransmission. Whether this happens is unclear. Local neurotoxicity with both ester and amide local anesthetics is extremely rare.[35] de Jong stated: "Negligible neurotoxicity is demonstrated by complete recovery of function after regional nerve block, as well as by light microscopic studies. Neural damage may, however, be produced by non–drug-related physical actions."[36] For example, intraneural injection of a peripheral nerve will produce damage secondary to compression ischemia. See table 3–3.

Skeletal muscle may be more sensitive than nerve tissue to local anesthetics.[37] Denervation-like change in skeletal muscle has been noted more

Table 3–3. Potential peridural neurologic concerns with HIV infection

CNS	HIV infection
	↑ Intracranial pressure from a tumor
	Local anesthetic systemic toxicity
PNS	Guillain-Barré syndrome
	Local anesthetic neural toxicity
	Epidural catheter neural injury or exacerbation of neural disease
	Vacuolar myelopathy
	Intraneural injection injury

with the potent, long-acting drug bupivacaine than with the less potent, short-acting drug lidocaine.[38] These changes are completely reversible by muscle regeneration within two weeks. Since interaction of local anesthetic with skeletal muscle would be more likely after peripheral nerve blocks than with spinal or epidural anesthesia, this is of little clinical importance in this context.

Could the physical presence of the epidural catheter produce or exacerbate neurologic disease? In an article on regional analgesia for patients with chronic neurologic disease, Crawford and colleagues concluded that epidural catheters or local anesthetics do not influence the progress of disease.[39] In a 1985 report Steiner and colleagues questioned epidural catheterization of four patients in whom Guillain-Barré syndrome chronologically followed epidural anesthesia by one to two weeks;[40] however, in three of the four patients one other common trigger of Guillain-Barré syndrome was present (pregnancy in one, surgery in two). In only one of the four cases did they cite the local anesthetic used. Subsequently, in 1986, Rosenfeld and colleagues reported the successful use of morphine sulfate, given in boluses over 10 days by epidural catheter, in a patient with Guillain-Barré.[41] While noting extreme vigilance for any changes in the patient's neurologic status, they found a return to full neurologic function. In 1987 McGrady reported the case of a woman two weeks postdiagnosis of Guillain-Barré syndrome who was managed during labor, cesarean section, and postoperatively with epidural bupivacaine and who recovered without ventilatory support at any stage.[42] Epidural anesthesia was chosen to avoid any respiratory depressant drugs during her labor and cesarean section; no apparent after-effects were attributed to the epidural. Most recently, in 1989, Gautier and cohorts reported Guillain-Barré syndrome 24 hours after an obstetrical epidural anesthetic, but they concluded that a causal relationship with the demyelinating process was unlikely because of the unusually fast onset of symptoms.[43] As mentioned in chapter 6, a case was reported (T. Janisse, C. Loar, P.P. Raj, "Pain of Guillain-Barré Syndrome Treated with Continuous Epidural Local Anesthetic," unpublished data, 1990) of an epidural bupivacaine infusion to relieve dysesthetic pain in a man with

Guillain-Barré syndrome. The patient's symptoms improved dramatically, and no exacerbation of his neurologic disease was found.

Certainly, increased intracranial pressure from a tumor would be an absolute contraindication to a peridural anesthetic. The CSF fluid volume or pressure could be significantly altered by the addition of local anesthetic used for spinal anesthesia. Dural puncture, either to deliver a spinal anesthetic or as a complication of an epidural injection or catheter placement, may result in a fluid leak that could alter CSF pressure or volume dynamics. The result could be catastrophic brainstem herniation.

HIV encephalopathy is more commonly associated with subcortical brain atrophy and demyelinative lesions in the periventricular white matter. These are less likely to result in a decreased CSF compartment or increased CSF pressure. Early clinical manifestations of HIV encephalopathy, as mentioned earlier, include cognitive, behavioral, and motor symptoms. Of more concern at this point may be whether a person so afflicted can give informed consent and will be able to cooperate during a regional anesthetic, and in face of these potential problems, whether a regional anesthetic will be less harmful than a general anesthetic that could potentiate already abnormal CNS function. Studies in the aged after general anesthesia have demonstrated prolonged recovery of psychomotor and cognitive skills.[44] A person with HIV encephalopathy may have less CNS reserve or reduced neuronal function, as may a geriatric person, which may result in slowed recovery from general anesthesia. Peripheral concerns with peridural anesthesia may be less important than CNS concerns with general anesthesia.

Up to 20% of AIDS patients eventually develop vacuolar degeneration of the spinal cord associated with paresis, ataxia, and incontinence.[45,46] If an HIV-infected patient were to receive a spinal or epidural anesthetic and these neurological complications were to occur later due to the disease, the cause might be attributed to the anesthetic. Before performing either of these major regional techniques, therefore, this point should be specifically covered with the HIV-positive patient and properly documented on the chart when informed consent is being sought.

In summary, when contemplating a regional anesthetic, concern about local anesthetic neurotoxicity may be minimal compared to the fear of neurologic complication implicating the regional anesthetic, a difficult case to disprove. This should not dissuade anesthesiologists, however, since neurotoxicity is so rare. Skeletal muscle is more sensitive than nerve tissue to long-acting local anesthetics, and the effects are completely reversible. Epidural catheter exacerbation of neurologic disease is controversial, but recent studies support a lack of causal relationship. If a person with HIV encephalopathy can give informed consent, a regional anesthetic would offer maximum benefit with minimum CNS impact. A person with AIDS and evidence of vacuolar myelopathy presents a dilemma solved only by evaluating the extent of spinal cord versus CNS disease.

Coagulation

[47]Anemia and thrombocytopenia[48] are often seen in patients with AIDS because of either the underlying disease[49] or the effects of chemotherapy. Thrombocytopenia surely affects one's decision whether to perform a regional or a general technique. A patient with a depressed platelet count may be a poor candidate for an epidural or a spinal due to increased risk of an epidural hematoma.

The answer is not absolute when questioning the safety of spinal or epidural anesthesia when coagulation abnormalities exist. With major abnormalities it is unsafe; with minor abnormalities it is controversial. People with HIV infection may have a wide range of coagulation changes, from subtle subclinical abnormalities and normal coagulation testing to clinically overt bleeding or abnormal testing. To evaluate the risk from coagulation abnormalities in a person with HIV infection, the anesthesiologist must know the current standard of practice and the coagulation abnormalities demonstrated by recent studies of HIV persons.

In a recent review article, Owens and colleagues noted that in a combined series of 50,000 spinal anesthetics no case of spinal hematoma was reported.[50] In the 33 reported cases of spinal hematoma with neurologic dysfunction after lumbar puncture, they found 79% had hemostatic abnormality—thrombocytopenia or use of anticoagulants or antiplatelet agents. Only six cases involved lumbar puncture for an anesthetic. In five of these it was difficult or bloody.

There have been four studies in which anticoagulation preceded or followed a spinal or epidural anesthetic (see table 3–4). No spinal hematomas or neurologic complications were reported. In the first study Matthews and Abrams[51] performed a lumbar puncture on 40 people to deliver intrathecal morphine for openheart surgery; 50 minutes later they were heparinized. In the second study Rao and El–Etr[52] reported on 4,011 people who had either continuous spinal or epidural anesthesia for peripheral vascular surgery and postoperatively. One hour after the anesthetic, heparin was given to increase the activated clotting time to twice baseline (less than 200 seconds). This

Table 3–4. Studies of peridural anesthetics with anticoagulation

Author	No. studied	Technique	Conditions
Matthews and Abrams	40	Single spinal	Heparinized for cardiopulmonary bypass
Rao and El-Etr	4,011	Continuous spinal or epidural	Heparinized for peripheral vascular surgery—intra- and postoperatively
Odoom and Sih	950	Epidural	Preoperative coumadin anticoagulation; heparinized for vascular surgery
Waldman et al.	56 (336 blocks)	Caudal	Anticoagulation: PT or aPTT 1.5 × control; or platelets <50,000

dosage was repeated every 6 hours, and the catheter was left in place for 24 hours postoperatively and removed just before a scheduled dose. In the third study Odoom and Sih[53] reported on 950 people taking oral anticoagulants, whose preoperative thrombotest was 19% (normal: 70%–130%). An epidural catheter was placed for vascular surgery, during which time subjects were heparinized. In the fourth study Waldman and colleagues[54] administered 336 caudal blocks with morphine and bupivacaine to patients with cancer who were either conticoagulated or thrombocytopenic from radiation or chemo-therapy. The prothrombin time (PT) or activated partial thromboplastin time (aPTT) was greater than 1.5 times control. The platelet count was less than 50,000. No spinal hematomas or neurologic complications were reported in any of these four studies.

Hematologic abnormalities have been reported in persons with HIV infection. In a study of 925 patients at risk for HIV disease, Costello found that thrombocytopenia was present in 2% of those who were HIV positive and in 15% of those with ARC or AIDS.[55] Initially, Zon and cohorts reported that one-third of AIDS patients studied had thrombocytopenia.[56] In their recent study thrombocytopenia was found in 13% of 8 asymptomatic people with HIV, 11% of 19 with ARC, and 33% of 45 with AIDS.[57]

Thrombocytopenia is not necessarily a progressive phenomenon. In those with AIDS active infection or drug therapy may be associated with a lower incidence of thrombocytopenia. Zon suggested that this may represent a reactive thrombocytosis. In addition, those asymptomatic people who develop AIDS may normalize their platelet counts, possibly due to defective clearance.[58]

A plasma anticoagulant may be present in people with AIDS. In a study group of 50, Cohen and colleagues reported an anticoagulant in 10; all had a prolonged activated partial thromboplastin time, and three also had a prolonged prothrombin time secondary to a mild factor II deficiency.[59] No other specific coagulation factor deficiencies were found. These and other tests were consistent with the coagulation studies of a lupus anticoagulant antibody.

In summary, a spinal hematoma with neurologic dysfunction is rare from any abnormality of the coagulation system: platelet, anticoagulant, or vasculature. Even spontaneous hemorrhage of unknown etiology and trau-matic punctures rarely cause a spinal hematoma. The exact level of platelet dysfunction or anticoagulation for safe administration of a spinal or epidural anesthetic is controversial. However, recent studies suggest that a mild degree of anticoagulation, thrombocytopenia, or platelet dysfunction does not increase the risk of spinal bleeding and hematoma formation if caution and appropriate timing are used for lumbar puncture or epidural catheter placement and removal, and in monitoring the level of anticoagulation. The increased practice of performing an epidural blood patch without complica-tions encourages anesthesiologists. Injection of up to 20 ml of blood into the epidural space to treat a dural puncture headache gives a perspective on the effects of excess blood in the epidural space. The injection may proceed until the side effect of increased back pain from spinal root pressure occurs. This demonstrates that producing a significant increase in epidural pressure does not necessarily result in complications.

Several additional points are important to remember:

1. The commonly used drugs that prolong the bleeding time are aspirin, antidepressants, antibiotics, local anesthetics, nitroglycerine, diuretics, beta blockers, and calcium channel blockers.
2. Heparin activity has been shown to vary with circadian rhythm; minimum aPTT values are noted in the morning, while maximum values are noted at night.[60]
3. Cooke et al. studied coagulation response to heparin and found it unpredictable.[61] In half of patients receiving 5,000 units of subcutaneous heparin, systemic anticoagulation occurred for up to four hours. The intent was to merely provide prophylactic blood levels of heparin.
4. Mini-dose prophylactic heparin does not produce systemic anticoagulation nor alter coagulation measurements. Low doses of heparin inhibit factor IXa and prolong only the aPTT. Large doses of heparin also inhibit factors Xa and IIa, prolonging both aPTT and PT and fully anticoagulating the patient.

Human immunodeficiency virus infection is associated with thrombocytopenia in up to 30% of people with AIDS and may be present in those who are asymptomatic. Asymtomatic people who develop AIDS may normalize their platelet counts. Coagulation may also be impaired by a lupus anticoagulant antibody.

Recommendations in persons with potential bleeding
1. Exclude any patients on anticoagulant therapy who also have blood dyscrasias, thrombocytopenia, leukemias, hemophilia, or abnormal liver function. The combination is an absolute contraindication.[52]
2. Test the coagulation response to heparin before performing a spinal or epidural procedure.[62] When clinically indicated, measure the aPTT for minidose heparin evaluation; the aPTT and PT for both low and large doses of heparin; the activated clotting time (ACT) for intraoperative heparin management; the Ivy bleeding time (IBT) for antiplatelet medications; and the PT, aPTT, IBT, and platelet level in the person with HIV infection, who may have a lupus anticoagulant or thrombocytopenia. See table 3–5.
3. Although the following do not contraindicate a spinal or epidural anesthetic, caution is advised: One arm of the coagulation system is impaired (PT or aPTT up to 1.5 times control, or ACT up to twice baseline level), platelet dysfunction (prolonged bleeding time), or thrombocy-

Table 3–5. Tests to define coagulation abnormalities

State	Test	Findings
Aspirin/other antiplatelet drugs	IBT	Increased (6–14 minutes)[63]
	Plts	Normal (>100,000)
Minidose heparin	aPTT	Normal (32–46 seconds)
	PT	Normal (11–16 seconds)
	ACT	<100 seconds
Low-dose heparin	aPTT	Increased (60–90 seconds)
	PT	Normal
	ACT	<200 seconds
Large-dose heparin	aPTT	Increased
	PT	Increased
	ACT	300–500 seconds
Coumadin	aPTT	Normal
	PT	Increased
HIV positive	IBT	Normal (1–9 minutes) or increased
	Plts	Normal or decreased
AIDS with a lupus anticoagulant	aPTT	Increased
	PT	Normal or increased
	Plts	Normal or decreased

topenia between 50,000 and 100,000. What is significantly less acceptable is to impair both arms of the coagulation factor system, or to impair one arm and have decreased platelet number or dysfunction, or to have decreased platelet number and dysfunction.

4. As one encounters or produces a greater degree of anticoagulation or platelet abnormality, developing a strong indication for a spinal or epidural anesthetic becomes increasingly important. The balance of risks and benefits must be carefully assessed, discussed with the patient, and documented in the medical record.

5. Performance of the lumbar puncture or epidural catheter placement must include a scrupulously sterile and meticulous technique by the most skilled and experienced anesthesiologist using a midline approach to avoid epidural veins. An epidural catheter without a stylet in the end must be inserted gently and only up to 3 cm. The dural puncture or catheter placement must be inserted more than 50 minutes prior to heparinization, and the catheter should be left in place until the lowest heparin activity occurs, possibly just before the next scheduled dose if one cannot wait for normalization of the coagulation system.

6. If frank blood is aspirated from an epidural catheter at any time during the procedure the technique should be abandoned and surgery delayed for 24 hours and then performed under general anesthesia.[50]

7. The patient must be monitored, closely, with special attention for early signs of prolonged, severe back pain, local tenderness, or neurological symptoms or signs. Should they occur, immediate neurosurgical consulta-

Table 3-6. Protocol for peridural access when potential bleeding

1. Exclude patients with contraindications.
2. Perform coagulation tests indicated.
3. Assess acceptability of abnormalities.
4. Weigh risks versus benefits with the patient.
5. Perform a skilled, cautious procedure.
6. If bloody, cancel for 24 hours; then give a general anesthetic.
7. Monitor closely; manage complications aggressively.

tion is necessary to evaluate the need for an emergency laminectomy and spinal decompression. A delay greater than 12 hours could result in irreversible neurologic damage, including paralysis or urinary or fecal incontinence. See table 3-6.

SAFETY CONSIDERATIONS

Blood transfusions

The blood pool in the United States has been much safer since 1985, when the testing for HIV antibodies was started. Recent estimates show that 5 to 25 infectious units of blood per million mistakenly pass the screen and are given to patients.[64,65] The reasons are lack of test sensitivity, blood donors that are infected but not seroconverted, and clerical errors in releasing screened blood known to be HIV positive.

Since blood and blood products cannot be guranteed to be HIV-free, they should be given only as necessary. The anesthesiologist would be well-advised to consult with the surgeon before proceeding with a transfusion and to note their joint decision to give blood, together with the clinical indication, on the anesthetic record.

The use of autologous blood to prevent HIV infection is common now and is highly advised. On the other hand, the use of the directed donations by friends and family members has little virtue. Sometimes, under pressure by patients or families to get such a donation, persons with an unrevealed risk factor such as IV drug abuse or homosexuality will donate to keep their secret hidden.

Transmission of HIV to health care workers[66,67]

Patients rarely pass HIV to health care workers, but in a handful of cases this has happened, usually when a dirty needle was being recapped or manipulated in some fashion. The probability of acquiring an HIV infection after such an injury is about 0.5%.[67] In very few cases have health care workers seroconverted after their skin or mucous membranes contacted blood from an HIV-infected patient; the chance of such infection is probably a great deal less than 1%. Nevertheless, any part of the body that becomes contaminated with the bodily fluids of any patient should be immediately and thoroughly washed.

All hospitals now follow a protocol after such an accident. New protocols are being developed to treat the health care worker preventively, before seroconversion, should such a mishap come about. Currently, the National Institute of Health (NIH) is studing the use of prophylactic azidothymidine in this connection.[68]

Many accidents can be prevented by the use of protective garb any time that contact with the bodily fluid of any patient can be expected. Gloves are generally sufficient, but gowns, masks, and eye coverings are recommended depending on the extent of exposure possible in a particular case. To prevent the need for mouth-to-mouth resuscitation, ambu bags, airways, and other such emergency airway equipment should be liberally dispensed throughout the hospital wherever its use seems likely to arise.

Special care should be taken with the treatment of critically ill emergency room patients who come to surgery.[69] Up to 16% of patients from socially disadvantaged areas who are suffering from severe trauma have been found to be HIV-positive. They are often bleeding profusely and require numerous invasive procedures—endotracheal intubation, arterial puncture, intravenous catheter placement, and so forth. In their haste to stabilize these patients medical personnel tend to dispense with protective clothing even during major resuscitations. In the second of two studies from Johns Hopkins Hospital, when 333 people were known to have AIDS in Baltimore, Kelen and co-workers found that 6% of 2,544 consecutive patients had HIV infection.[70] Of those who gave a history of a recent negative HIV test, 15% had unrecognized HIV infection. The health providers followed universal precautions during only 44% of all interventions and in only 19% of interventions for profuse bleeding. "The most common reasons given by providers were insufficient time to put on protective attire and interference with procedural skills." Kelen reported.

Since most cases of HIV transmission to health care workers result from cuts or nicks with sharp, contaminated objects, these professionals must be very careful with such items. Needles should not be recapped, bent, broken, removed from the syringe, or manipulated by hand in any other manner. The entire needle-syringe unit should be discarded into a large puncture-resistant container located nearby (not down the hall). Containers should never become so filled that they cannot hold these contaminated objects with ease.

Although HIV can live several days outside the human body even after dry, it is unlikely to pose much threat to the properly attired anesthesiologist. A solution of either 70% alcohol or household bleach diluted 1 to 10 in water kills the virus in less than a minute.[71] A variety of agents used routinely for disinfecting the operating room should perform adequately,[72-74] although perhaps less rapidly than alcohol or bleach. The labels of these products should be consulted concerning their potency against HIV. Exposure to ethylene oxide and steam in the process of sterilization readily kills this virus as well.

Reusable anesthetic items that touch mucous membranes should receive high-level disinfection. These items include laryngoscope blades, temperature probes, and fiberoptic scopes, all of which often become contaminated with blood. The use of disposable equipment minimizes the time and cost associated with suitable disinfection and prevents any concern about adequate cleanliness.

No healthy person has ever acquired an HIV infection, so it is believed, by the coughing or sneezing of an infected person. Saliva and sputum contain much less virus than an equal volume of blood. Still, one might prefer to extubate a patient with an HIV infection in the operating room rather than in the recovery room. In the former area all personnel are protectively clothed and the area itself undergoes daily thorough decontamination.

Although aerosolized sputum is probably not very dangerous, these authors find the aerosolized blood arising in a pink fog, breath by breath, from the chest of some patients undergoing thoracotomy to be much more worrisome. Other surgery, particularly involving high-speed power tools as used in orthopedics, can generate blood aerosols as well. Whether the usual face masks worn in the operating room are sufficient to prevent the inhalation of these mists needs to be studied. The use of two face masks might be considered until a definitive answer is available. Eye protection for these cases certainly seems advisable.

Transmission of HIV alone is not the only concern in the operating room. Since so many patients with AIDS have a concurrent cytomegalovirus infection, pregnant women are advised to avoid such exposure. The acquisition of certain other opportunistic organisms such as *Pneumocystis carinii* is less threatening because they require a severely depressed immune system to mount a successful infection.

The question often arises about contamination of the anesthesia machine by HIV-infected patients. There is no evidence that anyone has ever received an HIV infection from an anesthetic machine. Whether such trasmission is possible is not known, but it is probably very unlikely as HIV is not thought to be spread by the respiratory route. The concern remains however, that the opportunistic organism *Mycobacterium tuberculosis*, which may be present in 10% of AIDS patients, might be passed in this manner. The virility of this organism is high; a single bacterium is enough to initiate an infection. The routine use of a bacterial filter between the mask (and later between the endotracheal tube) and the circle system should be protective. The extra dead space of this device may create a sensation of smothering in some awake patients who are being preoxygenated. The practitioner who wants both a high level of protection for the machine and a minimum amount of dead space may wish to use two in-line bacterial filters, one in each of the two legs of the circle system.

The widespread hospital doctrine promulgated by the Centers for Disease Control known as "universal precautions" deals with those safeguards intended for use with all patients, regardless of their HIV status.[67] The underlying notion is that since many more patients are infected with HIV than the health care worker knows about, the sorts of precautions outlined in this section should be carried out for all patients.

Precautions always have an associated cost, whether it be the actual cost to the hospital of extra gloves or the inconvenience to the anesthesiologist of wearing extra protective clothing. "Universal precautions" represent a compromise between safety and these various costs and certainly provide a greater degree of safety than the usual procedures of only a year or two ago. They are widely used in part because they are neither too onerous to put up with nor too expensive to implement, even when applied to every single patient. They do the job of protection pretty well but certainly not in the best manner possible. At times the "universal precautions" are upgraded when new features concerning HIV become known.

If an anesthesiologist chooses to take special safety precautions, such as double-gloving or using a disposable circle system complete with soda lime, in the belief it is needed for a particular patient, he or she should be allowed to do so. Too often precautions in excess of the bare-bones "universal precatuions" are met with opposition from an infection control officer. The usual argument is that these practitioners are lulling themselves into a false sense of security since they encounter many equally infectious but undetected HIV-positive patients. Still, a patient known to be HIV-positive is known to be infectious and is certainly more dangerous than the average patient. Extra caution with such a patient is far from illogical, for by Sutton's Law "that's where the money is."

Furthermore, the impression that all patients infected with HIV are equally infectious is likely to be wrong.[75] It is useful to think of three different periods in the natural history of AIDS in this regard. Early in the disease, before antibodies have been produced, some patients may be especially infective. Rarely will the anesthesiologist be aware of such an infection; most pass unnoticed.

During the intermediate phase of infection, which usually lasts for years, the patient mounts and maintains a partially protective antibody response. These cases represent the majority of those infected patients whose disease is not yet recognized. Owing to their large number, it is especially fortunate that they may be less infectious than patients in the early stage of their infection.

Finally, as HIV continues its inexorable ravage of the immune system, the level of protective antibodies becomes too low to hold the infection in check. Free viral antigen, unbound to antibodies and in increasing amounts, signifies an ominous progression of the HIV infection.[76–78] During these last stages the patient often develops ARC and then AIDS and is thought to again become especially infectious due to an increased amount of free virus in bodily fluids.[75] Certainly, "universal precautions" must be vigorously applied to these patients, most of whom at this stage can be identified as infected; indeed, extra caution is clearly not unreasonable.

CONCLUSION

The elucidation of several dramatic presentations of HIV infection, such as grand mal seizure, syncope, Guillain–Barré syndrome, and hallucinations, underscores the importance of awareness and early diagnosis of this disease. It is not enough to await the progression to AIDS to become concerned about viral transmission and pathophysiologic abnormalities.

Anesthetic considerations must include knowledge of autonomic nervous system dysfunction in asymptomatic people, alteration in both peripheral nerve and muscle function, the potential for seizures, the possible presence of aseptic meningitis or HIV encephalopathy, and the potential for increased CNS sensitivity to opioids and hypnosedatives.

Most significant are the regional anesthetic implictions of HIV infection. Viral presence in the CSF of asymptomatic people intensifies transmission concerns when performing spinal and epidural blocks. A regional anesthetic may be preferable in a person with HIV encephalopathy, despite concern over the rare epidural abscess, and in the face of immunosuppression or systemic bacterial infection.

Concerns regarding possible exacerbation of neurologic disease by local anesthetic neurotoxicity or neural damage by placement of an epidural catheter, although theoretically inviting, are unfounded.

Coagulation abnormalities, including thrombocytopenia, platelet dysfunction, and an anticoagulant antibody, can be subclinical and defined only by testing, and the result may influence the anesthetic plan. A study–based approach to potential coagulation problems has been offered.

With new knowledge of and increasing experience with HIV infection, improved recognition, diagnosis, treatment, and management is possible. It is hoped that these will bring vital benefit to people.

In light of the present state of knowledge, the guidelines offered here seem reasonable, if perhaps conservative. Clearly, much remains to be learned about disease states resulting from infection with HIV that will be helpful to anesthesiologists in their care of patients.

This disease has no cure. Prevention, always important, becomes vital under these circumstances. Yet the danger to the anesthesiologist should not be exaggerated. HIV is not highly contagious; simple barrier protection with gloves and other appropriate apparel is effective against it. With reasonable care, an anesthesiologist can effectively treat these unfortunate persons and run very little risk of accidentally acquiring their infection.

REFERENCES

1. Greene ER, Jr: Spinal and epidural anesthesia in patients with the acquired immunodeficiency syndrome. Anesth Analg 65:1089–1093, 1986.
2. Prinscott J: Anesthetic consideration in a patient with acquired immune deficiency syndrome. MEJ Anesth 8(4):339–344, 1986.
3. Greene ER, Jr: Acquired immunodeficiency syndrome: An overview for anesthesiologists. Anesth Analg 65:1054–1058, 1986.

4. Kunkel SE, Warner MA: Human T-cell lymphotropic virus type III (HTLV-III) infection: How it can affect you, your patients, and your anesthesia practice. Anesthesiology 66:195–207, 1987.
5. Rankin JA, Collman R, Daniele RP: Acquired immune deficiency syndrome and the lung. Chest 94(1):155–164, 1988.
6. Murray JF, Garay SM, Hopewell PC, et al: Pulmonary complications of the acquired immunodeficiency syndrome: An update. Am Rev Respir Dis 135:504–509, 1987.
7. Peters SG, Prakash UBS: Pneumocystis carinii pneumonia. Am J Med 82:73–78,1987.
8. Brenner M, Ognibene FP, Lack EE, et al: Prognostic factors and life expectancy of patients with acquired immunodeficiency syndrome and Pneumocystis carinii pneumonia. Am Rev Respir Dis 136:1199–1206, 1987.
9. Kales CP, Murren JR, Torres RA, et al: Early predictors of in-hospital mortality for Pneumocystis carinii pneumonia in the acquired immunodeficiency syndrome. Arch Intern Med 147:1413–1417, 1987.
10. Ruben FL, Talamo TS: Secondary pulmonary alveolar proteinosis occurring in two patients with acquired immune deficiency syndrome. Am J Med 80:1187–1190, 1986.
11. Garay SM, Belenko M, Fazzini E, et al: Pulmonary manifestations of Kaposi's sarcoma. Chest 91(1):39–43, 1987.
12. Meduri GU, Stover DE, Lee M: Pulmonary Kaposi's sarcoma in the acquired immune deficiency syndrome. Am J Med 81:11–18, 1986.
13. Wallace JM, Hannah J: Cytomegalovirus pneumonitis in patients with AIDS. Chest 92:198–203, 1987.
14. Wasser L, Talavera W: Pulmonary crytococcosis in AIDS. Chest 92:692–695, 1987.
15. Morris JC, Rosen MJ, Marchevsky A, et al: Lymphocytic interstitial pneumonia in patients at risk for the acquired immune deficiency syndrome. Chest 91(1):63–67, 1987.
16. Johnson PC, Khardori N, Najjar AF, et al: Progressive disseminated histoplasmosis in patients with acquired immunodeficiency syndrome. Am J Med 85:152–158, 1988.
17. Cohen IS, Anderson DW, Virmani R, et al: Congestive cardiomyopathy in association with the acquired immunodeficiency syndrome. N Engl J Med 315:628–630, 1986.
18. Calabrese LH, Proffitt MR, Yen-Lieberman B, et al: Congestive cardiomyopathy and illness related to the acquired immunodeficiency syndrome (AIDS) associated with isolation of retrovirus from myocardium. Ann Intern Med 107:691–692, 1987.
19. Evenhouse M, Haas E, Snell E, et al: Hypotension in infection with the human immunodeficiency virus. Ann Int Med 107(4):598–599, 1987.
20. Elder G, Dalaka M, Pezeshkpour G, et al: Ataxic neuropathy due to ganglioneuronitis after probable acute human immunodeficiency virus infection. Lancet 2:1275–1276, 1986.
21. Eidelberg D, Sotrel A, Vogel H, et al: Progressive polyradiculopathy in acquired immune deficiency syndrome. Neurology 36:912–916, 1986.
22. Hollander H, Stringari S: Human immunodeficiency virus-associated meningitis. Am J Med 83:813–816, 1987.
23. So YT, Holtzman DM, Abrams DI, et al: Peripheral neuropathy associated with acquired immunodeficiency syndrome. Arch Neurol 45:945–948, 1988.
24. Cheung TW, Weg I: The implications of human immunodeficiency virus (HIV) infection and accidental falls (AF) among young patients in a city hospital. Vih International Conference on AIDS, Montreal, Abs.# MBP198, 1989.
25. Robinson G, Wilson SE, Williams RA: Surgery in patients with acquired immunodeficiency syndrome. Arch Surg 122:170–175, 1987.
26. Konotey-Ahulu FID: Surgery and risk of AIDS in HIV-positive patients. Lancet 2:1146, 1987.
27. Thomson DA: Anesthesia and the immune system. JBCR 8(6):483–487, 1987.
28. Bruce D, Wingard DW, Anesthesia and the immune response. Anesthesiology 34:271–282, 1971.
29. Salo M: Effects of anaesthesia and surgery on the immune reponse. In: Watkins J, Salo M (eds) Trauma, Stress and Immunity in Anaesthesia and Surgery. London: Butterworth Scientific, pp 211–253, 1982.
30. Jubert AV, Lee ET, Hersh EM, et al: Effects of surgery, anesthesia and intraoperative blood loss on immunocompetence. J. Surg Res 15:399–403, 1973.
31. Baker AS, Ojemann RG, Swartz MN, Richardson EP: Spinal epidural abscess. N Engl J Med

293:463, 1975.
32. Hancock DO: A study of 49 patients with acute spinal extradural abscess. Paraplegia 10:285, 1973.
33. Treacy M, Lai L, Costello C, Clark A: Peripheral blood and bone marow abnormalities in patients with HIV related disease Br J Hameatol, 65:289–294, 1987.
34. Zon LI, Groopman JE: Hematologic manifestations of the human immunodeficiency virus (HIV). Semin Hematol 25(3):208–218, 1988.
35. Skou JC: Local anesthetics II: The toxic potencies of some local anesthetics and of butyl alcohol, determined on peripheral nerve. Acta Pharmacol Toxicol 10:292, 1954.
36. de Jong RH: Local anesthetics. In: Raj PP (ed) Practical Management of Pain. Chicago: Year Book Medical Publishers, 539–556, 1986.
37. Covino BG: Clinical pharmacology of local anesthetic agents. In: Cousins MJ (ed) Neural Blockade in Clinical Anesthesia and Management of Pain. Sydney: J.B. Lippincott, 111–145, 1988.
38. Libelius R, Sonnesson B, Stamenovic BA, Thesleff S: Denervation–like changes in skeletal muscle after treatment with a local anesthetic (Marcaine). J Anat 106:297, 1970.
39. Crawford JS, James FM, Nolte H, et al: Regional analgesia for patients with chronic neurologic disease and similar conditions. Anaesthesia 36:821–822, 1981.
40. Steiner I, Argov Z, Cahan C, et al: Gillain–Barré syndrome after epidural anesthesia: Direct nerve root demage may trigger disease. Neurology 35:1473–1475, 1985.
41. Rosenfeld B, Borel C, Hanley D: Epidural morphine treatment of pain in Guillain–Barré syndrome. Arch Neurol 43:1194–1196, 1986.
42. McGrady EM: Management of labour and delivery in a patient with Guillain–Barré syndrome (letter). Anaesthesia 42:899, 1987.
43. Gautier PE, Pierre PA, Van Obbergh LJ, Van Steenberge, A: Guillain–Barré syndrome after obstetrical epidural analgesia. Reg Anesth 14(5):251–512, 1989.
44. Shafer A, White PF: Anaesthesia for outpatient surgery. In: Nunn JF, Utting JE, Brown BR, Jr (eds) General Anaesthesia, 5. Woburn, MA: Butterworth 1018–1035, 1989.
45. Ho DD, Rota TR, Schooley RT, et al: Isolation of HTLV-III from cerebrospinal fluid and neural tissues of patients with neurologic syndromes related to the acquired immunodeficiency syndrome. N Engl J Med 313:1493–1497, 1985.
46. Petito CK, Navia BA, Cho E-S, et al: Vacuolar myelopathy pathologically resembling subacute combined degeneration in patients with the acquired immunodeficiency syndrome. N Engl J Med 312:874–879, 1985.
47. Puppo F, Torresin A, Lotti G, et al: Autoimmune hemolytic anemia and human immunodeficiency virus (HIV) infection. Ann Intern Med 109(3):249–250, 1988.
48. Leaf AN, Laubenstein LJ, Raphael B, et al: Thrombotic thrombocytopenic purpura associated with human immundeficiency virus type 1 (HIV-1) infection. Ann Intern Med 109(3):194–197, 1988.
49. Stella CC, Ganser A, Hoelzer D: Defective in vitro growth of the hemopoietic progenitor cells in the acquired immunodeficiency syndrome. J Clin Invest 80:286–293, 1987.
50. Owens EL, Kasten GW, Hessel EA: Spinal subarachnoid hematoma after lumbar puncture and heparinization: A case report, review of the literature, and discussion of anesthetic implications. Anesth Analg 65:1201–1207, 1986.
51. Matthews ET, Abrams LD: Intrathecal morphine in open heart surgery. Lancet 2:543, 1980.
52. Rao TLK, El-Etr AA: Anticoagulation following placement of epidural and subarachnoid catheters: An evaluation of neurologic sequelae. Anestheslology 55:618–620, 1981.
53. Odoom JA, Sih IL: Epidural analgesia and anticoagulant therapy: Experience with one thousand cases of continuous epidurals. Anaesthesia 38:254–259, 1983.
54. Waldman SD, Feldstein GS, Waldman HJ, et al: Caudal administration of morphine sulfate in anticoagulated and thrombocytopenic patients. Anesth Analg 66:267–268, 1987.
55. Costello C: Haematological abnormalities in human immunodeficiency virus (HIV) disease. J Clin Path 41:711–15, 1988.
56. Zon LI, Arkin C, Groopman JE: Haematologic manifestations of the human immunodeficiency virus (HIV). Br J Haematol 66:251–256, 1987.
57. Zon LI, Groopman JE: Haematologic manifestations of the human immune deficiency virus (HIV). Semin Hematol 25(3):208–218, 1988.

58. Walsh C, Krigel R, Lennette E, et al: Thrombocytopenia in homosexual patients: Prognosis, response to therapy, and prevalence of antibody to the retrovirus associated with the acquired immunodeficiency syndrome. Ann Intern Med 10:542, 1985.
59. Cohen AJ, Philips TM, Kessler CM: Circulating coagulation inhibitors in the acquired immunodeficiency syndrome. Ann Intern Med 104:175, 1986.
60. Decousus HA, Croze M, Levi FA, et al: Circadian changes in anticoagulant effect of heparin infused at a constant rate. Br J Med 290:341–344, 1985.
61. Cooke ED, Lloyd MJ, Bowcock SA, Pilcher MD: Monitoring during low-dose heparin prophylaxsis. N Engl J Med 294:293–294, 1976.
62. Eichhorn JH: Spinal anesthesia and anticoagulant therapy. JAMA 262(3):411, 1989.
63. Hertzendorf LR, Stehling LC, Davey FR: Comparison of bleeding times performed on the arm and the leg. Am J Clin Pathol 87:393–936, 1987.
64. Peterman TA, Lui K-J, Lawerence DN, et al: Estimating the risks of transfusion-associated acquired immune deficiency syndrome and human immunodeficiency virus infection. Transfusion 27:371–374, 1987.
65. Ward JW, Holmberg SD, Allen JR, et al: Transmission of human immunodeficiency virus (HIV) by blood transfusions screened as negative for HIV antibody. N Eng J Med 318(8):473–478,1988.
66. Centers for Disease Control. Recommendations for prevention of HIV transmission in health-care settings. MMWR 36(suppl no. 2S), 1987.
67. Centers for Disease Control. Update: Universal precautions for prevention of transmission of human immunodeficiency virus, hepatitis B virus, and other bloodborne pathogens in health-care settings. MMWR 37:377–388, 1988.
68. NIH will offer AZT to employees exposed to HIV; U.S. Medicine April 1989, p 1.
69 Baker JL, Kelen GD, Sivertson KT, et al: Unsuspected human immunodeficiency virus in critically ill emergency patients. JAMA 257(19):2609–2611, 1987.
70. Kelen GD, DiGiovanna T, Bisson L, et al: Human immunodeficiency virus infection in emergency department patients. JAMA 262(4):516–522, 1989.
71. Resnick L, Veren K, Salahuddin SZ, et al: Stability and inactivation of HTLV-III/LAV under clinical and laboratory environments. JAMA 255(14):1887–1891, 1986.
72. Quinnan GV, Wells MA, Wittek AE, et al: Inactivation of human T-cell lymphotropic virus, type III by heat, chemicals, and irradiation. Transfusion 26:481–483, 1986.
73. Goldenheim PD: Inactivation of HIV by povidone-iodine. JAMA 257(18):2434, 1987.
74. Editoral: Disinfecting HTLV-III easily accomplished with standard reagents. Infect Dis Alert 4:93, 1985.
75. Redfield RR, Burke DS: HIV infection: The clinical picture. Sci Am 259(4):90–98, 1988.
76. Phair JP: Human immunodeficiency virus antigenemia. JAMA 258(9):1218, 1987.
77. Pedersen C, Nielsen CM, Vestergaard BF, et al: Temporal relation of antigenaemia and loss of antibodies to core antigens to development of clinical disease in HIV infection. Br Med J 295:567–569, 1987.
78. deWolf F, Goudsmit J, Paul DA, et al: Risk of AIDS related complex and AIDS in homosexual men with persistent HIV antigenaemia. Br Med J 295:569–572, 1987.

4. MANAGEMENT OF THE PARTURIENT WITH AIDS

M. JOANNE DOUGLAS

Since the recognition of acquired immunodeficiency syndrome (AIDS) as a disease complex in the early 1980s, it has rapidly assumed the proportions of an epidemic.[1,2] With the failure to discover an effective treatment, morbidity and mortality from this single disease entity will continue to increase. The primary event is infection with a retrovirus, human immunodeficiency virus (HIV), of which two specific types, type 1 and 2, are known. HIV specifically attacks the T4 lymphocytes, helper T4 cells, leading to their depletion. This depletion seriously impairs the body's ability to defend itself against infection by viruses, fungi, parasites, and some bacteria.[2] HIV is transmitted through semen, blood, breast milk, and, to a lesser degree, other body fluids.[3]

The major groups at risk from HIV infection are the sexually active and the intravenous drug abusers. While initially seen in male homosexuals, the crossover into the heterosexual population has occurred secondary to heterosexual contact with a person at risk from AIDS and to the sharing of needles in those who are intravenous drug abusers. Heterosexual transmission is now the leading cause of HIV infection in the world,[4] while in North America intravenous drug abuse is the main route.[5,6] Those who have received blood and blood products are another group at risk.[7] Hemophiliacs and their spouses were at high risk through this method of transmission, although better screening methods and awareness, with subsequent restraint in the use of blood products, has lessened this risk.

WOMEN AND AIDS

Masur and colleagues reported in 1982 on the presence of opportunistic infection in previously healthy women, suggesting that these cases might be related to those seen in males.[8] Following that report several reports have appeared on AIDS in women.[9-12]

Twenty-six percent of heterosexual AIDS patients in the United States are women.[10] In Africa the majority of transmission is through heterosexual contact, while in North America the primary route of infection is through intravenous drug abuse, with heterosexual transmission through intercourse with an infected male currently playing a secondary role.[13] With time this secondary route may assume greater importance, especially in the adolescent female. Education has not yet had an impact on this group, as shown in a study conducted in Boston in 1987.[14] In that study 200 adolescent females were asked a series of seven questions related to sexual activity: number of partners, condom use, history of sexually transmitted diseases (STDs), source of knowledge about AIDS, concerns with respect to AIDS, and their future sexual activity. This study pointed out the lack of awareness of heterosexual transmission (the belief being that it occurred only in homosexual males), the failure to obtain the male partner's history of high-risk behavior, and the lack of condom use. In a group of 21 subjects who had an STD, only 3 used condoms.

WOMEN, PREGNANCY, AND AIDS

The majority of women infected with HIV are in the childbearing years. The impact of this disease in relation to pregnancy and perinatal transmission is currently being studied.[15-21] In 1984 Rawlinson and colleagues presented the first report of AIDS in pregnancy—a case of disseminated Kaposi's sarcoma.[22] However, a maternal death possibly attributable to AIDS, although not confirmed, was reported by Wetli and co-workers in 1983.[23] This was a case of Listeria sepsis in a Haitian woman who died 3½ hours after giving birth. This maternal mortality report was followed by others, including Jensen et al., in 1984,[24] and Minkoff et al., in 1986.[25]

Debate continues about the effect of AIDS on pregnancy and, conversely, of pregnancy on the course of AIDS.[21] Initial reports suggested an increase in premature rupture of the membranes, premature labor, and intrauterine growth retardation.[18] These reports were retrospective, and further studies have now suggested that most of the differences previously seen could be attributed to poor antenatal care and nutrition in both intravenous drug abusers and those from a poor socioeconomic background.[16,20]

Pregnancy has been thought to accelerate the course of AIDS. Retrospective studies by Scott and colleagues[26] and by Minkoff[27] demonstrated a more rapid progression to overt disease in postpartum, HIV-postivie females. In contrast, in a study of congenital HIV infection in the Bahamas, only one of 18 mothers died of a complication possibly related to AIDS.[20] Some of the women had as many as three subsequent pregnancies and, although their children may have died, they remained asymptomatic.

Proposed factors leading to progression include ongoing intravenous drug abuse, continued exposure to an HIV–infected partner, presence of concurrent infections (herpes simplex virus [HSV], cytomegalovirus [CMV], human papilloma virus [HPV]), and the "immunosuppressive" effect of pregnancy.[29]

Transplacental transmission is thought to occur in the first trimester of pregnancy. Evidence for this exists in the reports of an HIV embryopathy,[30] recovery of viral antigen in the thymus of a preterm baby born by cesarean section to a woman with AIDS,[31] and recovery of virus from fetuses obtained at therapeutic abortion.[32] Additionally, the virus could be acquired during vaginal birth, as it has been isolated from cervical secretions, although evidence supporting this means of transmission has not yet been found. HIV has been isolated from breast milk, thus breast feeding is not recommended in HIV–positive women.[33]

Follow-up on children born to HIV–positive women shows varying rates of disease development.[15–18] The European Collaborative study[16] followed 100 babies for up to 15 months or until death from AIDS or AIDS-related complex. Of these 100 children 24 (24%) were presumed to be infected with HIV. Due to difficulties in diagnosing HIV infection in babies, this estimate may be low. All babies born to HIV–infected mothers will be antibody positive at birth due to passive transmission of the antibody and may remain positive for up to 15 months. Another confounding variable is that the babies could test antibody negative as AIDS develops.

ANESTHESIA AND AIDS IN THE PARTURIENT

To date much of the literature on this subject has dealt with preventing transmission of AIDS to the anesthesiologist, rather than focusing on the problem of AIDS patients and, in particular, the AIDS parturient. Practitioners must address some of the issues to consider when determining the best form of anesthesia/analgesia for these patients. To estimate the current numbers of pregnant AIDS patients being anesthetized, a group of obstetric anesthesiologists from the United States, Canada, and the United Kingdom were surveyed while attending the annual meeting of the Society for Obstetric Anesthesia and Perinatology in Seattle in May 1989. See table 4–1.

The results of this questionnaire (limited though it is) point out several dilemmas facing the practicing anesthesiologist. First, 78% of obstetric anesthesiologists have not anesthetized pregnant AIDS patients, and 39% have not administered anesthesia to known HIV–positive pregnant patients. Second, those who have anesthetized pregnant AIDS patients have limited experience: 71% have anesthetized less than 5 patients, with only one having anesthetized 10–20 patients. Obviously, anesthesiologists from some of the

Table 4–1. Results of 1989 Society for Obstetric Anesthesia and Perinatology (SOAP) survey on AIDS and obstetric anesthesia

---

DEMOGRAPHIC DATA
1. Number of questionnaires handed out: 300
2. Number completed: 122
3. Number of deliveries per year in their hospital:

<1000	3	2%
1000–3000	40	33%
3000–5000	47	39%
>5000	32	26%

QUESTIONS ASKED
1. Number HIV-positive pregnant patients anesthetized January–May 1989?

0	48	39%
<10	58	48%
10–20	11	9%
>20	5	4%

2. Would they administer a regional anesthetic to an HIV-positive pregnant patient?

Yes	111	91%
No	6	5%
No answer	2	2%
Would depend	3	2%

3. Number of pregnant patients with clinical AIDS anesthetized?

0	94	77%
0–5	20	16%
5–10	7	6%
10–20	1	1%
>20	0	

4. Would they administer a regional anesthetic to a pregnant patient with clinical AIDS?

Yes	81	66%
No	22	18%
No answer	3	3%
Uncertain	9	7%
If no contra-indications	7	6%

ANESTHESIA FOR PARTURIENT WITH CLINICAL AIDS
1. Number of replies   22
2. Type of procedure

Labor	15	40%
C/S	15	40%
Other (TL, ?)	8	20%

3. Analgesia for labor

Regional	8	80%
IV	2	20%

4. Anesthesia for C/S

Regional	11	73%
General	4	27%
(One would use regional)		

5. Response to local anesthetics

Normal	22	100%
Abnormal	0	

---

major centers for AIDS patients were not represented by this survey. The third dilemma is that there are no published case reports or summaries of clinical experience dealing with the AIDS parturient. Finally, obvious differences exist with respect to the possible use of regional anesthesia for both labor and operative procedures. Of those who have anesthetized the AIDS parturient, 11% would not use regional anesthesia. These are the questions—what are the possible answers?

CONSIDERATIONS FOR ANESTHESIA

Factors to be considered when anesthetizing the parturient with AIDS include the disease itself, the type of procedure to be performed, and any treatment the patient may be undergoing.

AIDS: The disease entity

AIDS is a multisystem disease.[3] Those systems of particular interest to the anesthesiologist are the neurological, respiratory, and hematologic systems. Because the physiological changes of pregnancy profoundly affect these systems these factors must be considered before undertaking any anesthetic procedure.

Neurological system

AIDS affects both the central and peripheral nervous systems at any point in the course of the illness.[34,35] Frequently, neurological disease may be the presenting manifestation of HIV–related disease. AIDS–related central nervous system disease includes primary HIV syndromes (encephalopathy, aseptic meningitis, vacuolar myelopathy), opportunistic viral illnesses (cytomegalovirus, herpes simplex types I and II, herpes varicella–zoster virus, papovavirus), nonviral infections (toxoplasmosis, cryptococcus, candida), neoplasms (primary CNS lymphoma, metastic systemic lymphoma, and metastatic Kaposi's sarcoma), and cerebrovascular disorders (infarction, hemorrhage, and vasculitis).[36] Other central nervous system disorders are less frequent. Diseases of the peripheral nervous system and myopathies are also seen.[37,38] Acute and subacute-chronic polyneuropathies, mononeuritis multiplex, and demyelinating and inflammatory changes have been found. The cases of myopathy are similar to polymyositis. Further, a peripheral neuropathy, called predominantly sensory neuropathy, has been found in AIDS and AIDS-related complex patients[39] that appears to be associated with the late manifestations of HIV infection. Recent estimates of the incidence of neuropathy or myopathy are clinical occurrence in 40% of infected adults, with pathological evidence in 80%.[35]

The implications of these factors for anesthesia include the dilemma of administering a regional anesthetic to patients with known neurological disease and to patients in whom neurological disease may progress or develop.[40]

Respiratory system

Pneumocystis carinii pneumonia (PCP) has been responsible for much of the morbidity and mortality associated with AIDS. With the prophylactic use of pentamidine, PCP is declining in frequency, but other opportunistic pulmonary infections are taking its place.

Pregnancy leads to altered pulmonary mechanics and blood gas changes and predisposes the patient to hypoxemia. The added problem of a disease that can affect the respiratory system increases the risk of hypoxia for these patients.

Hematologic system

Anemia, leukopenia, and idiopathic thrombocytopenia have all been reported in these patients. Since many of them are also intravenous drug abusers, or have been chronically ill and required intravenous antibiotics, it may also prove technically difficult to cannulate peripheral veins for anesthetic and intravenous fluid administration.

General comments

These patients frequently are very ill. Many of them are wasted and may be febrile. Routine hemoglobin, platelet count, and coagulation profile should be obtained. Additionally, electrolytes (specifically potassium) and arterial blood gases should be known prior to anesthetic administration. With significant wasting and/or myopathy, use of muscle relaxants will have to be carefully monitored; if a regional technique is selected, ventilation should be assessed. The use of pulse oximetry in these patients is essential.

Treatment of AIDS

The therapy for AIDS is undergoing rapid change. The current standby is 3'azidothymidine (AZT, Zidovudine).[41,42] This drug has antireverse transcriptase activity with effects on DNA, and patients may therefore present for termination of pregnancy. There is considerable debate about maintaining patients on AZT if they become pregnant.[43] Azidothymidine is known to cross the blood–brain barrier and thus will also cross the placenta.[44] Whether this transmission might confer benefit in preventing transmission of HIV to the fetus or might cause congenital abnormalities is unknown. Azidothymidine therapy is associated with bone marrow suppression and myopathy, diseases that may lead to cessation of therapy. Patients on AZT therapy should be screened for hematologic and electrolyte abnormalities prior to receiving anesthesia.

Type of anesthesia: Regional vs. general

As noted earlier, there is some question as to whether regional anesthesia should be used in these patients.[40] Certainly, in the face of an obvious contraindication, such as coagulopathy, sepsis, or severe hemorrhage, few would choose a regional technique. Some anesthesiologists may rule out a regional anesthetic based on concerns with respect to (1) introducing a pathogen into the central nervous system, (2) administering a regional anesthetic to patients likely to develop neurological symptoms that are usually progressive, and (3) availability of an alternative technique. Certainly, retrospective studies have not demonstrated any introduction of the herpes viruses into the central nervous system when a regional technique was used in the infected patient, so this fear may prove similarly unwarranted.[45,46]

In labor, alternative forms of analgesia (parenteral narcotics, inhalational agents, ketamine) may not prove so attractive. The difficulty in obtaining adequate pain relief without possible impairment of maternal and neonatal ventilation is one factor against narcotic use. Additionally, many of these patients are chronic drug abusers and some may require an excessive narcotic dosage. Ketamine administration to patients with possible central nervous system pathology, particularly encephalopathy, may also be fraught with difficulties. Patient cooperation for any form of analgesia may be poor and may lead to technical difficulties.

These same dilemmas face the anesthesiologist considering the patient for cesarean section. Although no statistical data are yet available as to frequency of cesarean section in AIDS patients, there are several reasons for them to have an operative delivery. Many of these patients present with premature labor, with premature rupture of the membranes, or with an unstable lie, and so proceed to cesarean section. Additionally, they frequently have other STDs, such as herpes genitalis, that may make cesarean birth more common.

It is essential that the patient and anesthesiologist discuss the alternatives prior to a decision about the technique to be employed. If a regional method is used for either labor or delivery, it must be performed with strict aseptic technique. The patient should be considered immunocompromized. The most experienced practitioner should perform the epidural or spinal anesthetic, in order to lessen the number of attempts. Although beneficial for postoperative analgesia management, epidural morphine should possibly not be used. Suggestions of increased incidence of herpes simplex recrudescence in patients receiving epidural morphine[47–49] may contraindicate its use in the AIDS patient, possibly in the HIV–positive, asymptomatic patient. Viruses, such as cytomegalovirus, have been suggested as possible cofactors in the development of clinical AIDS.[50] If this should prove true, then anything that might lead to viral recrudescence should be avoided.

General anesthesia is also not without risk in these patients. Studies have indicated that it may have a role in suppressing the immune response.[51] Additionally, manipulation of the airway and ventilation/perfusion abnormalities in these patients may lead to intraoperative and/or postoperative hypoxia. Problems associated with the use of muscle relaxants and central nervous system depressants should also be considered, especially in the patient with overt neurological disease, myopathy, or severe wasting.

Provided that all of these factors are considered and discussed with the patient, patient choice will be one of the prime determinants of the technique employed. That these factors have been considered and discussed should be entered into the patient's chart, and these patients should be followed to note any complications.

The problem of pain

Recent information has emphasized the complex nature of pain and the importance of motivational, cognitive, emotional, and other psychological factors on the individual's total pain experience.[52,53] In no other area do these factors play as great a role as in labor. The pain of labor has been equated to that of an amputated digit or of chronic back pain.[54] During labor the patient with AIDS may experience many emotions that may affect her pain. These could include guilt, for possibly bearing an affected child; fear, not only for herself but for her child; anger, for the position that she is in; and finally, an acute awareness of pain, secondary to previous experience with pain, possibly related to her disease. Many of these patients also suffer from the stigma of the disease and may have little or no support during labor. Others will be extremely ill and may find all procedures, including blood pressure measurement, painful.

No data have yet been published as to the quality of the labor pain experienced by these patients or to their response to various analgesics. The SOAP survey indicated that these patients had a labor experience similar to that of non HIV–infected women. These results, however, may be biased due to the anesthesiologists' reluctance to become involved with these seriously ill patients. These care-givers must be careful not to deny these patients adequate pain relief due to concerns of the health personnel.

Precautions for the anesthesiologist

Much has been written on the need for anesthesiologists to take precautions when anesthetizing any patient and, in particular, those who are HIV positive.[55–60] These precautions include barrier protection with gloves, gown, and goggles. Particular attention must be paid to handling sharp articles, needles, and scalpel blades that may be contaminated with blood containing HIV. Recapping of needles is a hazardous process. Anesthesiologists should attend to the disposal of all sharp objects in a puncture-proof container prior to removing their gloves. All need to develop the technique of cannulating veins and arteries while wearing gloves; gloves should also be worn for all procedures about the mouth (intubation, insertion of an oral airway, suctioning).

Protection of other patients must also be undertaken. Disposable anesthetic equipment should be used whenever possible. If nondisposable items must be used, they must be sterilized appropriately at the conclusion of each case.

SUMMARY

The latest information worldwide indicates that there are now 154,667 patients with AIDS (WHO, May 1, 1989). Of this number approximately 5% to 7% are women, most in the childbearing age. Prenatal testing for HIV infection has been advocated in those patients with self-identified risk factors.[61,62] Such testing would help in the subsequent management of these patients and help identify when counseling should be offered. However, because studies have shown that many seropositive women do not admit to risk factors, all health personnel should consider all patients as potentially HIV positive and take appropriate precautions for themselves and for other patients. This is particularly true in the delivery suite, where additional hazards in the form of blood and amniotic fluid exist.

The anesthetic management of the parturient with AIDS is complex. Consideration must be given not only to the patient, to provide her and her fetus with the best analgesia/anesthesia with the least risk of complications, but also to the anesthesiologist and other health personnel to provide them with protection from possible transmission of HIV. As anesthesiologists become more involved with the care of the AIDS parturient, they will be better able to determine the best possible management.

REFERENCES

1. Quinn TC, Zacarias FRK, St. John RK: AIDS in the Americas—An emerging public health crisis. N Engl J Med 320:1005–1007, 1989.
2. Gallo RC, Montagnier L: AIDS in 1988. Sci Am, 259:41–48, 1988.
3. Redfield RR, Burke DS: HIV infection: The clinical picture. Sci Am 90–98, October 1988.
4. Mann JM, Chin J, Piot P, et al: The international epidemiology of AIDS. Sci Am, 82–89, October 1988.
5. Heyward WL, Curran JW: The epidemiology of AIDS in the U.S. Sci Am, 72–81, October 1988.
6. Leads from the MMWR: Acquired immunodeficiency syndrome associated with intravenous-drug use—United States, 1988. JAMA 261:2314–2316, 1989.
7. Curran JW, Lawerence DN, Jaffe H, et al: Acquired immunodeficiency syndrome (AIDS) associated with transfusions. N Engl J Med 310:69–75, 1984.
8. Masur H, Michelis MA, Wormser GP, et al: Opportunistic infection in previously healthy women—Initial manifestations of a community-acquired cellular immunodeficiency. Ann Intern Med 97:533–539, 1982.
9. Harris C, Small CB, Klein RS, et al: Immunodeficiency in female sexual partners of men with the acquired immunodeficiency syndrome. N Engl J Med 308:1181–1184, 1983.
10. Guinan ME, Hardy A: Epidemiology of AIDS in women in the United States (1981 through 1986). JAMA 257:2039–2042, 1987.
11. Johnson MA, Webster A: Human immunodeficiency virus infection in women. Br J Obstet Gynaecol 96:129–134, 1989.
12. Howard LC, Hawkins DA, Marwood R, et al: Transmission of human immunodeficiency virus by heterosexual contact with reference to antenatal screening. Br J Obstet Gynaecol 96:135–139, 1989.
13. Peterman TA, Cates W, Curran JW: The challenge of human immunodeficiency virus (HIV) and acquired immunodeficiency syndrome (AIDS) in women and children. Fertil Steril 49:571–581, 1988.

14. Grace E, Emans SJ, Woods ER: The impact of AIDS awareness on the adolescent female. Adolesc Pediatr Gynecol 2:40–42, 1989.
15. Rubinstein A, Sicklick M, Gupta A, et al: Acquired immunodeficiency with reversed T4/T8 ratios in infants born to promiscuous and drug-addicted mothers. JAMA 249:2350–2356, 1983.
16. The European Collaborative Study: Mother-to-child transmission of HIV infection. Lancet 2:1039–1043, 1988.
17. Italian Multicentre Study: Epidemiology, clinical features, and prognostic factors of paediatrc HIV infection. Lancet 2:1043–1045, 1988.
18. Minkoff H, Nanda D, Menez R, et al: Pregnancies resulting in infants with acquired immunodeficiency syndrome or AIDS-related complex: Follow-up of mothers, children, and subsequently born siblings. Obstet Gynecol 68:288–291, 1987.
19. Minkoff H, Nanda D, Menez, et al: Pregnancies resulting in infants with acquired immunodeficiency syndrome or AIDS-related complex. Obstet Gynecol 69:285–287, 1987.
20. Howard-Gardiner H, Roberts PD, Dunn PM: Congenital human immunodeficiency virus (HIV) infection in the Bahamas. Br J Obstet Gynaecol 96:140–143, 1989.
21. Gloeb DJ, O'Sullivan MJ, Efantis J: Human immunodeficiency virus infection in women I. The effect of human immunodeficiency virus on pregnancy. Am J Obstet Gynecol 159:756–761, 1988.
22. Rawlinson KF, Zubrow AB, Harris MA, et al: Disseminated Kaposi's sarcoma in pregancy: A manifestation of acquired immune deficiency syndrome. Obstet Gynecol 63:2S–6S, 1984.
23. Wetli CV, Roldan EO, Fojaco RM: Listeriosis as a cause of maternal death: An obstetric complication of the acquired immunodeficiency syndrome (AIDS). Am J Obstet Gynecol 147:7–9, 1983.
24. Jensen LP, O'Sullivan MJ, Gomez-del-Rio M, et al: Acquired immunodeficiency (AIDS) in pregnancy. Am J Obstet Gynecol 148:1145–1146, 1984.
25. Minkoff H, Haynes deRegt R, Landesman S, et al: Pneumocystis carinii pneumonia associated with acquired immunodeficiency syndrome in pregnancy: A report of three maternal deaths. Obstet Gynecol 67:284–287, 1986.
26. Scott GB, Fischl MA, Klimas N, et al: Mothers of infants with the acquired immunodeficiency syndrome. Evidence for both symptomatic and asymptomatic carriers. JAMA 253:363–366, 1985.
27. Minkoff HL: Care of pregnant women infected with human immunodeficiency virus. JAMA 258:2714–2717, 1987.
28. Minkoff HL, Nanda D, Menez R, et al: Follow-up of mothers of children with AIDS. Obstet Gynecol 87:288–291, 1987.
29. Quinn TC, Glasser D, Cannon RO, et al: Human immunodeficiency virus infection among patients attending clinics for sexually transmitted diseases. N Engl J Med 318:197–203, 1988.
30. Wiznia A, Marion R, Hutcheon G, et al: Further delineation of the HIV embryopathy (Abstract 7231) IVth International Conference on AIDS, Stockholm, 1988.
31. Lapointe N, Michaud J, Pekovic D, et al: Transplacental transmission of HTLV-III virus. N Eng J Med 312:1325–1326, 1985.
32. Eitelbach F, Unger M, Huang Z, et al: HIV-antigens can be demonstrated immunohistochemically in formalin-fixed material from therapeutic abortions of HIV-exposed pregnancies (Abstract MBP 18). Vth International Conference on AIDS, Montreal, Canada, 1989.
33. Ziegler JB, Cooper DA, Johnson RD: Postnatal transmission of AIDS-associated retrovirus from mother to infant. Lancet 1:896–898, 1985.
34. Dalakas M, Wichman A, Sever J: AIDS and the nervous system. JAMA 261:2396–2399, 1989.
35. Elder GA, Sever J: AIDS and neurological disorders: An overview. Ann Neurol 23(suppl)S4–S6, 1988.
36. Levy RM, Bredesen DE, Rosenblum ML: Opportunistic central nervous system pathology in patients with AIDS. Ann Neurol 23(suppl):S7–S12, 1988.
37. Parry GJ: Peripheral neuropathies associated with human immunodeficiency virus infection. Ann Neurol 23(suppl)S49–S53, 1988.
38. Dalakas MC, Pezeshkpour GH: Neuromuscular diseases associated with human immunodeficiency virus infection. Ann Neurol 23(suppl):S38–S48, 1988.
39. Cornblath DR, McArthur, JC: Predominantly sensory neuropathy in patients with AIDS and AIDS-related complex. Neurology 38:794–796, 1988.

40. Greene ER. Spinal and epidural anesthesia in patients with the acquired immunodeficiency syndrome (letter). Anesth Analg 65:1090–1091, 1986.
41. Hirsch MS: AIDS commentary—Azidothymidine. J Infect Dis 157:427–431, 1988.
42. Cload PA: A review of the pharmacokinetics of zidovudine in man. J of Inf 18:15–21, 1989.
43. Discussion of Symposium on Zidovudine, Mandal BK, Glover SC (eds). J of Inf 18:67–75, 1989.
44. Unadkat JD, Lopez-Anaya A, Schumann LA: Transplacental transfer of zidovudine (Abstract MBP). Vth International Conference on AIDS, Montreal, Canada, 1989.
45. Ramanathan S, Sheth R, Turndorf H: Anesthesia for cesarean section in patients with genital herpes infections: A retrospective study. Anesthesiology 64:807–809, 1986.
46. Crosby ET, Halpern SH, Rolbin SH: Epidural anesthesia for cesarean section in patients with active recurrent genital herpes simplex infections (Abstract D29). 21st Annual Meeting, Society for Obstetric Anesthesia and Perinatology, Seattle, 1989.
47. Douglas MJ, McMorland GH: Possible association of herpes simplex type I reactivation with epidural morphine administration (letter). Can J Anaesth 34:426–427, 1987.
48. Gieraerts R, Navalgund A, Vaes L, et al. Increased incidence of itching and herpes simplex in patients given epidural morphine after cesarean section. Anesth Analg 66:1321–1324, 1987.
49. Crone LL, Conly JM, Clark KM, et al: Recurrent herpes simplex virus labialis and the use of epidural morphine in obstetric patients. Anesth Analg 67:318–323, 1988.
50. Skolnik PR, Kosloff BR, Hirsch MS: Bidirectional interactions between human immunodeficiency virus type 1 and cytomegalovirus. J Infect Dis 157:508–514, 1988.
51. Hansbrugh JF, Zapata-Sirvent RL, Bartle EJ, et al: Alterations in splenic lymphocyte subpopulations and increased mortality from sepsis following anesthesia in mice. Anesthesiology 63:267–273, 1985.
52. Bonica JJ: Pain of parturition. Clinics in Anesthesiology 4:1 31, 1986.
53. Wuitchik M, Bakal D, Lipshitz J: The clinical significance of pain and cognitive activity in latent labor. Obstet Gynecol 73:35–42, 1989.
54. Melzack R: The myth of painless childbirth (John J. Bonica Lecture). Pain 19:321–337, 1984.
55. Davies JM, Thistlewood JM, Rolbin SH, Douglas MJ: Infections and the Parturient: Anesthetic considerations—AIDS and hepatitis: A guide for obstetrical anaesthetists. Can J Anaesth 35(3):270–277, 1988.
56. Greene ER: Acquired immunodeficiency syndrome: An overview for anesthesiologists. Anesth Analg 65:1054–1058, 1986.
57. Kunkel SE, Warner MA: Human T-cell lymphotropic virus type III (HTLV-III) infection: How it can affect you, your patients, and your anesthesia practice. Anesthesiology 66:195–207, 1987.
58. Arden J: Anesthetic management of patients with AIDS (letter). Anesthesiology 64:660–661, 1986.
59. Browne RA, Chernesky MA: Infectious diseases and the anaesthetist. Can J Anaesth 35:655–665, 1988.
60. Storniolo FR, Cheek TG, Shelley WC, et al: Acquired immunodeficiency syndrome. In: James FM, Wheeler AS, Dewan DM (eds) Obstetric Anesthesia: The Complicated Patient, 2nd ed. Philadelphia: FA Davis, pp 447–452, 1988.
61. Landesman S, Minkoff H, Holman S, et al: Seroprevalence of human immunodeficiency virus infection in parturients. Implications for human immunodeficiency virus testing programs of pregnant women. JAMA 258:2701–2703, 1987.
62. Minkoff HL, Holman S, Beller E, et al: Routinely offered prenatal HIV testing (letter). N Engl J Med 319:1018, 1988.

5. OROFACIAL PAIN IN AIDS PATIENTS

DOUGLAS W. ANDERSON AND MARSHALL D. BEDDER

Treating orofacial pain manifestations in the patient with acquired immuno-deficiency syndrome is a new challenge for algologists. Pain may precede definitive diagnosis or arise late in the progression of the disease. Current knowledge on specific entities is presented in the following sections to aid in the comprehensive care of the AIDS patient. A multidisciplinary approach is evolving in the effective control of pain-related problems.

Patients with acquired immunodeficiency syndrome frequently present with signs and symptoms referable to the head and neck.[1] New manifestations of this disease are being reported as awareness grows. Patients early in their disease may see a variety of health care professionals for pain complaints. Often, the dentist is the only health professional with regular contact, making diagnosis and treatment of oral lesions extremely important. Patients diagnosed with AIDS are now presenting to surgeons, internists, and pain specialists for treatment of their specific pain complaints. The manifestations of orofacial pain in the AIDS patient can be categorized as follows: oro-pharyngeal, cutaneous and lymph node/glandular. See table 5–1. Previous studies have demonstrated clinical evidence of head and neck disease in 40–50% of all AIDS patients.[2] This presentation may be the first and only clinically detectable evidence of the disease.[3] Computed tomography (CT) and Magnetic resonance imaging (MRI) techniques have been added to the conventional clinical examination—laryngoscopy or barium pharyngography —to further delineate the nature and extent of lesions.[4] CT and MR assessment guide biopsy and assist in treatment planning.

Table 5–1. Orofacial manifestations of AIDS

OROPHARYNGEAL
Aphthous ulcer
Oral candidosis
Hairy leukoplakia
Oral herpes simplex
Oral Kaposi's sarcoma
Periodontal disease
Purpuric gingivitis
Venereal warts
Oral squamous cell carcinoma
Necrotizing ulceration
Pharyngitis
Laryngeal granuloma

CUTANEOUS
Orofacial zoster
Perioral herpes simplex
Perioral cytomegalovirus
Perioral Kaposi's sarcoma
Facial nerve palsy
Neuralgia
Disseminated histoplasmosis

LYMPH NODE/GLANDULAR
Cervical lymph node enlargement
Intrasalivary node enlargement
Adenoidal enlargement
Tonsillar enlargement
Parotid enlargement

OROFACIAL ZOSTER VIRUS, HERPES SIMPLEX VIRUS, AND CYTOMEGALOVIRUS

Perioral herpesvirus infections, such as varicella-zoster virus, herpes simplex virus (HSU), and cytomegalovirus (CMV), are common early signs of symptomatic infection with human immunodeficiency virus.[3,5] Cytomegalovirus is disseminated in the AIDS population,[6–8] and the presence of Epstein-Barr virus (EBv) and Epstein-Barr virus DNA is also high in those who have AIDS or are at risk for AIDS.[8,9] Herpes simplex virus and varicella-zoster virus are less frequent in clinical occurrence,[8] but when they develop the lesions are painful and sometimes debilitating. Cytomegalovirus and Epstein-Barr virus may present as nonpainful, insidious infections. Lymphadenopathy, malaise, weight loss, generalized wasting, and occasional fever, which may be transient or prolonged, are characteristic. These viruses are associated with deficient cellular immunity and are considered a factor in the pathogenesis of the immunocompromised state, leading to life-threatening opportunistic infections.

In the general population, acute herpes simplex virus infection is the most common viral infection after the common cold. The virus resides only in cells of ectodermal origin. Two types of infection occur, characterized as primary and recurrent. Intraoral primary infection, affecting both children and adults, is characterized by the onset of fever, intraoral discomfort, and inflammation. Yellowish, fluid-filled vesicles appear, then rupture and ulcerate, leaving a grey membrane covering with an erythematous border. These vesicles usually measure less than one centimeter in diameter. Recurrent infections follow the same course usually seen in adults, even with a high antibody titer. Precipitating associative causes are thought to be trauma, fatigue, ultraviolet light exposure, anxiety, emotional upset, and respiratory infections. Recurrent infection is secondary to reactivation of the dormant virus residing in epithelial cells.[10] Diagnosis is made by Papanicolaou smear, although recent advances in monoclonal antibody testing, performed in two to three hours is more sensitive and specific for herpes simplex virus infection.[11] Visual diagnosis can sometimes be difficult if the lesions are secondarily infected with bacteria or fungus.

Herpes virus infections occur in approximately 90% of immunocompromised, bone-marrow-transplant recipients within two weeks of transplantation.[8] In homosexual men herpes simplex virus infections are common,[12,13] and in homosexual patients with AIDS fatal viremias can occur in spite of treatment.[14]

In the immunocompromised patient intraoral lesions predominantly occur in keratinized tissue.[15] The hard palate, attached gingiva, and alveolar ridge are common sites, as well as the tongue, mucosal surface of the lip, and the lip proper. The intraoral and perioral sites may progressively enlarge in those AIDS individuals who do not seek diagnosis and treatment for early infection. Although oral herpes simplex virus infections are a less common manifestation of AIDS,[16] the range of occurrence in homosexual men and AIDS patients is between 5% and 9%.[8,17,18]

Oral herpes simplex virus infections are painful. Proper diagnosis is essential to determine the appropriate treatment and sequence of drugs. Concurrent antibiotic and antifungal therapy should be administered when an overlying bacterial or candidal infection occurs. For herpes simplex virus infections in the immuncompromised patient, topical Idoxuridine or intravenous vidarabine (10 mg/kg body weight daily) can be effective.[15] In the AIDS patient as well, 5% topical Acyclovir applied to the intraoral lesions six times daily or oral tablets one to two grams daily are effective. More aggressive treatment should include intravenous administration of Acyclovir.[12] Two percent lidocaine gel applied topically can temporarily relieve painful symptoms.

KAPOSI'S SARCOMA

As outlined earlier, presentation in the head and neck region is frequently the first and only clinically detectable evidence of AIDS. In ten patients in whom the initial manifestation of AIDS-related malignancies occurred in the head and neck region, six were found to have Kaposi's sarcoma.[3] One patient presented with a pimplelike skin lesion of the neck while others had palatal or nodal involvement. Other larger studies report 35%–50% of patients with the cutaneous, oral, and pharyngeal lesions of Kaposi's sarcoma as the presenting head and neck manifestations of AIDS.[1] Kaposi's sarcoma in AIDS may assume a wide variety of clinical presentations, including macular, papular, or nodular forms. Skin lesions 0.5–2.0 cm in diameter are usually non-pruritic and painless; the color can be pink, dark red, blue, or purple.

Kaposi's sarcoma is the most prevalent of the oral neoplastic lesions in the HIV patient. Oral findings of Kaposi's sarcoma in males not on immunosuppressive therapy are pathognomonic of AIDS.[16] Oral Kaposi's sarcoma has been observed in upwards of 50% of AIDS patients examined[18,19]; however, many were referred from a clinic for patients with Kaposi's sarcoma at the School of Medicine, University of California, San Francisco. The authors suggest this could account for the high incidence. Another study observed that 18 of 110 male homosexuals with HIV infection demonstrated Kaposi's sarcoma. Sixteen of the 18 men manifested oral Kaposi's sarcoma.[17] If only the AIDS patients are considered in this study, representing 47 of 110 HIV-infected people, 34% demonstrated oral Kaposi's sarcoma.[17]

The most frequent site of appearance of oral Kaposi's sarcoma is the palate.[10,20] The gingiva, alveolar mucosa, tonsils, and buccal mucosa are less frequent sites of occurrence.[20] Early lesions may present as flat red or purple pigmented mucosa. Raised macular or nodular lesions precede the late tumor stage. The neoplastic nature is not always apparent in superfical biopsy specimens because Kaposi's sarcoma arises from subepithelial layers.[19] Obtaining a connective tissue layer should increase the certainty of a correct diagnosis.

Histologically, the early and late tumor stages differ.[20] In the early stage extravasated red cells, atypical vascular channels, eosinophilic bodies, hemosiderin deposits, and inflammatory cells are prominent. In the late tumor stage, spindle cell components and mitotic figures are prevalent with fewer inflammatory cells present. Kaposi's sarcoma tends to displace rather than invade adjacent tissue.[20] The histologic features seen in elderly men do not vary from those in homosexual men.[21] Patients predisposed to Kaposi's sarcoma in general may have less immune dysfunction than those patients who develop opportunistic infections as the first manifestations of AIDS.[22] A prospective group of high-risk patients was followed for a median of 12 months. In those who presented with unexplained oral candidiasis, the initial T4/T8 ratio was significantly less in those who developed life-threatening opportunistic infections than in those who did not.[23] The T4/T8 ratio, in another group of high-risk patients with opportunistic infections, was significantly lower when compared with the same population who had Kaposi's sarcoma as their sole clinical manifestation.[22]

Oral Kaposi's sarcoma is not painful. However, opportunistic infections superimposed on an enlarging tumor may cause pain, difficulty in mastication, swallowing, and a decrease in airway patency depending on the location or enlargement of the tumor. Treating the opportunistic infections, after a proper diagnosis has been made, will provide symptomatic relief of pain and discomfort. Occasionally, tooth pain, gingival recession, and bone loss, occurring where there is a purplish enlarged vascular appearing gingiva (suggestive of Kaposi's sarcoma), can also cause minor pain. In this instance, removing the tumorous tissue will usually provide symptomatic relief.

Intraoral treatment options are aimed at removing or reducing tumor size. Chemotherapy, radiation, or carbon dioxide laser removal on unattached gingiva can be used in some instances. Low-dose radiation therapy, approximately 150 rads for 10 days, is effective. Always of concern are secondary bone infections that can lead to osteomyelitis, presenting further painful complications.

NEUROLOGIC MANIFESTATIONS

Neurologic manifestations of HIV can be divided into direct effect of HIV and indirect effects such as autoimmune phenomena, tumors, and opportunistic infections. Herpes simplex virus is the most commonly seen viral infection, followed by cytomegalovirus, varicella-zoster viruses, and papovirus. Non-viral infections include cryptococcus neoformans, toxoplasma gondii, mycobacteria, and spirochetes. Hodgkin's lymphoma is the most common neoplasm involving the central nervous system, with Kaposi's sarcoma being less common.

Neurologic complications of AIDS are being reported with greater frequency; older reports show 37% of AIDS patients developing complications during their illness.[24] Schofferman stated that pain due to peripheral neuropathy is the most common pain in people with AIDS (PWA) with advanced disease.[25] This appears to be due to direct involvement of the nerve with HIV or CMV.[26] Impairment of craniofacial nerves has also been reported.[27] Two cases resulted from progressive multifocal leukoencephalopathy (PML). Hypesthesia, as well as facial paralysis, hemianopsia, and deafness was the clinical presentation.[28]

Progressive multifocal leukoencephalopathy is characterized by focal demyelinization with proliferation of capillaries and microglia cells and the presence of atypical astrocytes.[29] This CNS syndrome appears to result from cerebral infection with papovavirus.[30] The differential diagnosis for painful sensorimotor neuropathy should now include AIDS as well as diabetes, amyloidosis, nutritional deficiencies, and certain chemotherapeutic agents.

The response to treatment of painful sensory neuropathy in AIDS patients with tricyclic antidepressants appears to be mixed.[25,31,32] Partial symptomatic relief was experienced in 50% of patients in one series, while azidothymidine (AZT) provided no relief. Transcutaneous nerve stimulation may offer some symptomatic relief, although experience is limited.

One further neurological manifestation of AIDS may be headaches. The differential diagnosis of headaches in AIDS patients must be expanded to include:

1. Direct involvement of the brain with HIV or toxoplasmosis.
2. Cryptococcal meningoencephalitis.
3. Lymphoma of the brain.
4. Muscle tension headache.
5. Cervical disease.
6. Medication.

Treatment of headache pain would proceed with treatment of the underlying pathology if possible or with the traditional stepwise escalation of analgesics.

PAROTID ENLARGEMENT

Parotid enlargement due to benign lymphoepithelial lesion (BLL) and to benign hyperplastic lymphadenopathy similar to BLL[34] has been described. Benign lymphoepithelial lesion is a nodular or diffuse form of salivary gland enlargement. The parotid lymphadenopathy and the BLL syndrome have been described in intravenous drug users, and a causative relationship to HIV is suspected. A recent review outlined the differential diagnosis in parotid enlargement.[33] See table 5–2. Contrast material enhanced computed tomographic scans have been performed in patients at risk for AIDS and with facial swelling.[37] All scans revealed parotid cysts as well as diffuse homogeneous cervical adenopathy. There was a 92% correlation of parotid cysts at CT and positive antibodies to HIV. The CT scan was the first indication of seropositivity in three cases of the twelve studied. It has been recommended that patients who present with unilateral or bilateral parotid masses, and who are discovered on CT or MR scanning to have multiple parotid cysts and cervical lymph nodes suggestive of hyperplastic adenopathy, should be considered to have AIDS until it is proven otherwise.[38]

In patients with chronic bilateral parotid gland swelling, pain may be present in 78%.[39]

RECURRENT APHTHOUS STOMATITIS

In healthy persons recurrent aphthous stomatitis, referred to as recurrent aphthous ulcers, is a common form of lesion found in the oral environment. Its etiology is unknown, but an immunological mechanism is suggested.[40] The lesions are rounded, well–circumscribed ulcers with characteristic inflammatory, erythematous, marginal halo. They are self–limiting, rarely progress, and usually resolve within two weeks of appearance. They are painful and can be confused with trauma, bacterial infection, or malignancy. These lesions appear on non–keratinized tissue. Recurrent aphthous ulcers can occur in the immunocompetent patient.[41] In the AIDS patient intra– and extra–oral lesions can prevent proper nutritional intake due to associated pain. When the lesions

Table 5–2. Differential diagnosis of parotid enlargement

PAROTID GLAND	
BENIGN	PATHOLOGIC
Primary salivary gland tumor	Primary salivary gland tumor
Sebacious cysts	
Lipomas	
Fibromas	
Neurofibromas	
Lymphangiomas	
Diabetes mellitus[35]	
Anorexia nervosa[36]	
PAROTID GLAND LYMPH NODES (INTRAPAROTID AND PERIPAROTID)	
BENIGN	PATHOLOGIC
Tuberculosis	Metastatic carcinoma (oral primary)
Sarcoidosis	Scalp tumor (melanoma)
Mumps	Parotid tumor (lymphoma)
Measles	AIDS-related complex (ARC)

SOURCE: SHAHA ET AL.[33]

are major (more than 6 millimeters in diameter) normal oral function may be severely impaired. Although recurrent aphthous ulcers are a less common oral feature of AIDS patients,[5,16] there appears to be recurrence in male homosexuals. Decreased host resistence may be the cause.[10] In one study 8% of 375 homosexual males had aphthous/erythema multiform lesions. Reichart observed recurrent aphthous ulceration in 3 of 110 patients with HIV infection.[17]

When the diagnosis is uncertain, a biopsy or culture should be done. When no infectious cause is found, oral prednisone or intravenous methylprednisolone, if the extent and severtiy of the lesions warrant more aggressive therapy, should be considered in the empirical treatment.[42] The associated pain should diminish with resolution of the ulcerative lesions. Maintenance doses of corticosteroids may be required if there is recurrence of the aphthous ulcers during drug tapering.

ORAL CANDIDA INFECTIONS

The most common oral fungal infection seen in the AIDS patient is candidiasis, which may present with pain. In this population signs or symptoms may not be present, and, if cultures are positive for candida, the presumption that one is a carrier must be considered.[43] *Candida albicans* is the most frequent species present, but other species may also exist.[10,44]

Oral candidiasis may be divided into descriptive categories.[45] Others have used different descriptive categories:[17,46] (1) pseudomembranous or thrush, (2) atrophic, which includes angular chelitis, and (3) hyperplastic candidiasis or leukoplakia. Another descriptive type is a papillary variant.[17]

The lesions of pseudomembranous candidiasis, or thrush, appear as soft, white-creamy, slightly raised or elevated plaques, sometimes grossly resembling milk curds. They frequently occur on the buccal mucosa and the lateral aspect and dorsum of the tongue, as well as on the palate, gingiva, vestibule, and floor of the mouth. The elevated plaques are easily wiped off, sometimes leaving a raw bleeding surface.

The lesions of atrophic candidiasis are characterized as erythematous, sometimes erosive, and the oral mucosa appears atrophic. The lesions appear on the lateral border of the tongue, buccal mucosa, pharynx, gingiva, and lip. Angular cheilitis, a variant of atrophic candidiasis, appears as a fold or fissure in the corners of the mouth that collects saliva and usually becomes secondarily infected with bacteria. Most often the lesions appear in people who wear dentures and are due to an intraoral candidal infection requiring antimycotic and sometimes antibiotic treatment.

The lesions of hyperplastic candidiasis, sometimes referred to as leukoplakia, are white, firm, granular coated, adherent, and unstrippable. The lesions appear mostly on the lateral border and dorsum of the tongue, and less frequently on the buccal mucosa, gingiva, pharynx, and lip. The papillary variant appears as erythematous papillary nodules always located on the hard palate.[17]

Nonspecific local oral host defense factors are protective against candida infection. These include epithelial turnover, saliva, lysozyme, oral microbial interactions and competition, iron, salivary glycoproteins, lactiferrin, and lactoperoxidase.[45] Healthy individuals have antibodies to *Candida*,[45] but those with AIDS do not have a lymphocyte response to *Candida* antigen, and recurrent infections are frequent.[47]

Candida must adhere to mucosal surfaces and colonize to cause disease. The yeast form may be pathogenic, and when infection occurs the local environmental changes favor the filamentous form. Some predisposing factors that alter the oral environment and cause a candidal infection are antibiotic therapy, diabetes, immunocompromise and xerostomia, particularly radiation-induced xerostomia.[43] In the immunocompromised patient oral candidiasis leads to morbidity and can coexist with severe opportunistic, often fatal, infections.[47] Oral candidiasis in patients with AIDS is a marker of esophageal candidiasis, and if esophageal symptoms are not present after failed antimycotic intraoral therapy, endoscopy should indicate esophageal involvement.[48]

The diagnosis of oral candidiasis is made by examining cultures in a variety of media and/or material plaque smears, macerated and suspended on microscopic slides using 20% potassium hydroxide, showing the typical hyphae. The appearance of hyphae in large numbers helps differentiate candidiasis from other pathological conditions such as vesicular eruptive lesions, median rhomboid glossitis, bacterial infection, and neoplasia.

Candidiasis is classified as a common oral manifestation of AIDS and an opportunistic infection.[16] Of the patients at risk for AIDS who presented with unexplained oral candidiasis, 59% of those studied developed serious opportunistic infections.[23] *Candida* was the most common oral infection found in 375 homosexual males examined. Sixty-six percent were found to be culture-positive, and 92% of these patients had oral signs and symptoms.[18] Both clinical and culture-positive *Candida* infection occurred in 57% of those with opportunistic infections in a population of 53 homosexual men with Kaposi's sarcoma. Scrapings of hairy leukoplakia lesions in 71 of 140 immunosuppressed homosexual men demonstrated *Candida* by smear and culture.[49] In 27 of 36 subgingival sites sampled, *Candida albicans* was present in plaque smears, and this has led some to think that *Candida* may be associated with the severe peridontitis seen in the AIDS patient.[50] In 80% of 110 HIV-positive patients examined, oral smears were taken and 85% were positive for *Candida albicans*. Thirty-eight of the 68 patients, or 56% had oral symptoms.[51]

A myriad of pharmaceutical preparations are available for antifungal therapy. The choice and/or combination of drugs depends on a number of factors, including systemic involvement; extent of local, oral, or esophageal involvement; and extent of dental alveolar disease present. Topical amphotericin B is indicated for the treatment of cutaneous or mucocutaneous infections. The intravenous form is reserved for progressive, potentially fatal fungal infections. Ketoconazole tablets, 200 to 400 mg per day, may be used, but hepatotoxicity can be of concern. Baseline and frequent liver function tests should be done. Ketoconazole should be taken with food since dissolution in an acid media is essential for absorption. Nystatin extemporaneous oral suspension, which must be used immediately after mixing, does not contain dextrose (50% W/V) or preservatives as does the regular oral suspension. Either nystatin oral pesstille or vaginal tablets dissolved orally may be appropriate, but they do contain sucrose and lactose, respectively. Clortrimazole vaginal tablets contain lactose, and the oral troche dissolved orally five times a day contains dextrose. Miconozole nitrate vaginal suppositories are suspended in a hydrogenated vegetable oil and may be dissolved and given orally, if sugar substrates are of concern in the oral environment.

Recurrent intraoral candidal infections in the AIDS patient can and do occur. Treatment regimens may have to be empirical. Patient education and cooperation is important. Once candidal infections are cleared up, a thorough inspection of the mucosal tissue is essential since Kaposi's sarcoma may be a finding.

HAIRY LEUKOPLAKIA

Hairy leukoplakia is likely a viral-induced intraoral lesion found predominantly on the lateral border of the tongue. Its appearance may be smooth or corrugated with hairy projections, sometimes markedly folded. The folds run vertically along the lateral border of the tongue. Many lesions are asymptomatic and subtle, and others, if secondarily infected with *Candida*, can be uncomfortable and mildly sore. Biopsy is important to confirm a diagnosis if the appearance is subtle. The lesions do not rub off.

Hairy leukoplakia was observed in 19 of 110 patients: 17 of these were male homosexuals, and 2 were intravenous drug abusers. Fourteen of the 19 had AIDS, and 5 had ARC.[17] Further studies found a 28% incidence of hairy leukoplakia in a population of 375 homosexual males. Others reported observations of hairy leukoplakia in 27% (3 of 11) of HIV-seropositive homosexual males.[52]

Possible immunosuppression should be suspected when a diagnosis is confirmed.[18] Although initially observed in homosexual males, hairy leukoplakia has been observed in women—a transfusion recipient and a hemophiliac.[53] It is associated with human papillomavirus[54] and Epstein-Barr virus. A symbiosis is suggested between the human papillomavirus and EBV that infects the subepithelial layers. Only the antigens of human papillomavirus and EBV, and EBV itself, can be demonstrated.[55]

The normal strict regulation of EBV replication appears to be altered in the HIV-immunocompromised patient. The reduced number of Langerhans cells in the mucosa from a HIV infection may contribute to formation of hairy leukoplakia lesions. However, no HIV has been recovered from a hairy leukoplakia lesion.[49] The clinical finding of hairy leukoplakia is correlated with risk for developing AIDS. Forty-eight percent of 155 immunosuppressed homosexual men developed AIDS within 16 months, and 83% by 31 months, after diagnosis and follow-up for leukoplakia.[49]

Treatment consists of antifungal therapy to relieve acute symptoms. Hairy leukoplakia itself is asymptomatic. Carbon dioxide laser treatment may remove the lesions, but recurrence is a problem. Topical application with a cotton swab of .05% Retin-A solution once daily may be successful for removal. However, repeated applications are necessary as the lesions reappear.[55]

PERIODONTAL DISEASE

A dynamic balance exists between oral microflora and host defenses. Any shift in the relationship that allows opportunistic cultivation of oral flora may cause disease. Natural host defenses, such as metabolic, genetic, mucosal, gingival, and salivary components that inhibit bacterial adherence and growth, moderate this relationship.

Gingival disease is a subclassification of periodontal disease.[56] Gingivitis is inflammation of the gingival tissues primarily caused by bacterial activity. Oral bacteria colonize at the tooth surface and gingival margin. If not removed, the bacterial and food substrate mass, referred to as plaque, has pathogenic potential. The pathogenic potential of dental plaque can vary among individuals and from one tooth to another within an individual.[57] Other areas of gingival disease include manifestations of systemic disease and hormonal alteration, drug-associated, disease and other disease associated with pathologic and physiologic changes in gingival health. The prevalence of gingivitis in at least one localized intraoral site per individual is reportedly between 80% and 100% and is seen in all age groups.[56]

Untreated gingivitis usually precedes periodontitis. There are subclassifications of adult and juvenile periodontitis;[56] however, all involve extension of the inflammatory process into the soft tissues and bone supporting the teeth, resulting in the progressive destruction of the surrounding tissues. The gingival loss of attachment to the tooth allows formation of periodontal pockets that harbor further plaque accumulation inaccessible to tooth brushing.

Periodontal disease is treatable and/or controllable, but in a small number of cases teeth may be lost in spite of treatment. Periodontitis may be characterized by periods of active disease alternating with periods of remission and periodontal attachment repair. Inflammation can be localized to one or two teeth or generalized and affect many or all teeth. Since the pathologic changes that occur in the periodontium are multifactorial, however, the cyclic hypothesis of periodontal destruction needs further study.[57]

Measurement of the epithelial attachment level by probing in the gingival sulcus and by demonstrating radiographic and clinical changes in alveolar bone height are clinical methods to evaluate periodontal disease activity. Long-term regular and frequent plaque control methods are essential for maintaining a healthy periodontium.

ACUTE NECROTIZING ULCERATIVE GINGIVITIS

The diagnosis of acute necrotizing ulcerative gingivitis can be made by clinical observation. It is characterized by inflammation, ulceration, soreness, interproximal necrosis of the gingival papillae and occasional free gingival margin, and spontaneous bleeding on contact. A grey erythematous necrotic membrane overlies any normal appearance of the gingiva. Ulcerations tend to spread from a single focus and can involve adjacent gingival margins. A fetid breath odor is characteristic. Ancillary clinical features are lymphadenopathy and occasional fever and malaise.[58]

A general fusiform and spirochete character represents the predominant portion of an array of bacterial types that can be cultured.[59] There is a reduced PMN and lymphocyte responsiveness.[58] A stress-induced increase in corticosteroid levels may decrease leukocyte function. The increased cortisol levels may provide selective nutritional advantage to some bacterial species associated with acute necrotizing ulcerative gingivitis.[59]

Predisposing factors of this disease are thought to be poor physical condition, psychological stress, smoking, local trauma or preexisting inflammation, and poor oral hygiene.[58] Epidemiological studies correlate acute necrotizing ulcerative gingivitis with cytomegalovirus infections and seroconversion in industrialized and underdeveloped countries.[60] Also, decrease in both T-lymphocyte helper/suppressor ratio in cell-mediated immunity, and unresponsiveness to the mitogen con-A, occurs in both diseases.[60]

The T4/T8 ratio of five homosexual men in one study was 0.54, with a normal ratio of 2.0–3.0. The incidence of acute necrotizing ulcerative gingivitis in the total number of homosexual men studied was 9.4%, with a normal population incidence of 0.02% to 0.08%. A higher than normal cytomegalovirus viruria was demonstrated in homosexual men from a venereal disease clinic, and a high incidence of cytomegalovirus antibody was detected (94%) in these homosexual males compared to heterosexual males (54%).[6] The cause-and-effect relationship to acute necrotizing ulcerative gingivititis, which some term AIDS-virus-associated periodontitis,[50] is not known. However, reports of acute necrotizing ulcerative gingivitis in patients at risk for AIDS, in homosexuals, or in diangosed AIDS patients are increasing. One study documented 38 homosexual men with AIDS-virus-associated periodontitis and atypical gingivitis, described as gingival edema and erythema extending to the alveolar mucosa.[50] Head and neck examinations demonstrated 36% of 11 HIV-seropositive patients,[52] and 6% of 110 patients with HIV infection,[17] had acute necrotizing ulcerative gingivitis. Eleven percent of the latter group revealed rapid progressive periodontitis,[17] while 17% of 375 homosexual males examined in an oral medicine clinic had periodontitis.[18]

Many HIV-infected patients are unaware of any intraoral problem. Early on periodontal disease may be an incidental finding in HIV patients, many of whom are well nourished and previously had good dental care. However, periodontal disease progresses as HIV infection becomes more severe. Acute ulcerative necrotizing gingivitis is painful and is probably preceded by the atypical, less-painful gingivitis. Since these problems occur in an age group that enjoys good health, a thorough medical history and examination, diagnostic testing procedures and appropriate consultations[52] are important in diagnosing HIV-infected periodontal disease and acute necrotizing ulcerative gingivitis.

When the administration of antibiotics in AIDS patients is indicated, their primary care physician should be consulted. Many of these patients are already on antibiotics or have opportunistic infections. The severity of these infections could be altered by misappropriation of care. Classically, however, in healthy patients, oral penicillin and/or metronidazole[59] is used as adjunctive therapy to help control the acute gingival or periodontal infection or subdue the refractory nature of these infections. Debridement of subgingival or supra-gingival plaque is the primary approach to reducing painful symptoms and disease severity. No antibiotic has been shown to alter subgingival plaque as a definitive therapeutic measure if there has been inadequate root scaling, root planing, and poor home care.[50] Topically, 5 cc of 10% Betadine applied 3–4 times daily using a conventional irrigating syringe may be therapeutic.[50] However, Betadine solution is not an approved or normally recommended intraoral rinse. Caution, and a reasonable, predicted, therapeutic benefit should precede its continued use. Chronic use of hydrogen peroxide is not recommended since there is potential for adverse effects.[62] A prescription mouthwash solution of 0.12% chlorhexadine, Peridex, used twice daily may effectively control plaque and gingivitis.[63] The solution contains 11.6% alcohol with a pH of 5.5. Continued empirical usage of this chemical as adjunctive therapy may depend on intraoral symptoms, adverse effects, progressive disease state, and cost. Fluoride rinses are important for maximum effectiveness of each agent. Candidal overgrowth may also have to be treated simultaneously and may go unrecognized as a coinfection unless its presence is diagnosed.

If atypical gingivitis, acute necrotizing ulcerative gingivitis, or related periodontal disease is left untreated, opportunistic infections and/or underlying malignancies may go undetected. Progression to osteonecrosis or osteomyelitis does occur, and these infections may proceed to life-threatening situations.

ENDODONTIC AND TOOTH PERIAPICAL INFECTIONS

Tooth pulp pathosis ranges from inflammatory to pulpal necrosis. Clinically, reversible pulpitis, characterized by sensitivity to heat or cold stimulus, subsides after a period. Normal pulp physiology and function resume after, for example, a routine filling is placed. Irreversible pulpitis is a clinical condition that warrants root canal therapy. Degenerative changes occur within the pulp, resulting in pain symptoms of increased intensity and duration that are uncharacteristic of normal adjacent teeth. Occasionally after pulp stimulation, when heat or cold is applied to the offending tooth, the pain response takes several seconds or minutes to abate. Periapical bone inflammation, and the intense percussion sensitivity sometimes felt, or a deep throbbing ache in the alveolar bone, is suggestive of further extension of the pulpal degenerative process. Other than mechanical or chemical injury to a tooth pulp, bacterial invasion of the pulp may cause pulpal degeneration. Bacteria may gain access by migration through the dentin as occurs in dental caries. Disruption of pulpal blood supply by trauma, and resulting necrosis in the absence of bacteria, provides a good environment for colonization of anaerobic bacteria. Bacteremias or bacterial invasion from diseased periodontal tissues or bone facilitates infection.

Periapical lesions are direct extensions of pulpal pathosis in the absence of diagnosable periodontal disease, demonstrating destruction of the periapical tissues. The extent of the acute or chronic inflammation or spread of infection is unpredictable. Usually, immediate intervention with root canal therapy designed to remove the necrotic tissue and seal the root apex is sufficient to prevent further problems. Depending on the extent and severity of periapical bone destruction and pain, however, surgical drainage of the infected bone is required. Tooth extraction, trephenation, incision, and drainage or root apicoectomy are procedures that may accomplish this.

Dental treatment in the AIDS patient is not contraindicated. Conservative therapy that produces the most effective treatment with the least risk to the patient should be considered. Root canal therapy is not contraindicated provided that the conventional orthograde approach relieves all symptoms and that radiographic evidence does not suggest further chronic extension of periodontal and/or bone destruction. Surgical intervention in AIDS patients, except tooth extraction or very necessary incision and drainage of an intraoral abscess, may be contraindicated. Osteomyelitis is a risk in immunocompromised and AIDS patients when endodontic root surgery is considered for the elective retention of a tooth after root canal therapy.

A variant in the spectrum of atypical facial pain, or pain of unknown origin, has been seen in our clinic in healthy, not-at-risk patients. Referred facial pain may be caused by tooth periapical inflammation or infection resulting in maxillary sinus dehisence before or after endodontic procedures. This referred pain may be diagnosed as atypical facial pain. The patient's sinus involvment and/or facial pain is refractory to treatment until the offending tooth is treated or extracted. A tooth origin for the pain and maxillary sinus symptoms are always found. Although the authors have not seen this in AIDS patients, unilateral maxillary sinus symptoms, excluding nasal and paranasal sinus pathology or opportunistic infection, may arise from an odontogenic source. With severe periodontal destruction or tooth abscess, the need for tooth extraction instead of root canal therapy is more obvious.

When tooth extraction is contemplated in the AIDS patient, the potential for a protracted healing course exists. In four patients who had dental extractions or osteotomies for impacted teeth, the average T4/T8 ratio was 0.4 and wound healing was protracted.[17] Palliative treatment of a postextraction osteitis is no different in the AIDS patient than in healthy patients. Packing of the extraction site with surgical, iodine-impregnated gauze strip, with frequent dressing changes, is recommended. Systemic antibiotics may have to be administered for several weeks. These are painful experiences that, if treated diligently, may be prevented from progressing to a more severe problem.

LARYNGEAL LESIONS

Laryngeal lesions can cause dysphagia, odynophagia, or hoarseness. Kaposi's sarcoma may involve the laryngeal mucosa as well as the more common pharyngeal location.[64] Sooy reported two cases of vocal cord paralysis, one secondary to vinca alkaloids and the other of unknown etiology.[24] A tracheostomy was required for an AIDS patient with multiple recurrent neck abscesses and laryngeal granuloma. Laser laryngoscopy is indicated for isolated lesions, and radiation therapy or chemotherapy is the treatment of choice for more extensive disease.

CONCLUSION

A multidisciplinary approach to treating orofacial pain in the AIDS patient is essential. From the specific topics presented in this chapter, the inexperienced practitioner may realize the complex set of pain problems that must be addressed simultaneously during treatment. For the experienced practitioner, we have attempted to present a body of information that is useful in the overall approach to treatment of the AIDS patient.

REFERENCES

1. Marcusen DC, Sooy CD: Otolaryngologic and head and neck manifestations of acquired immunodeficiency syndrome (AIDS). Laryngoscope 95(4):401–405, 1985.
2. Rosenberg RA, Schneider KL, Cohen NL: Head and neck presentations of acquired immunodeficiency syndrome. Otolaryngol Head Neck Surg 93(6):700–705, 1985.
3. Helsper J, Formenti S, Levine A: Initial manifestation of acquired immunodeficiency syndrome in the head and neck region. Am J Surg 152(4):403–406, 1986.
4. Olsen WL, Jeffrey RB Jr., Sooy CD, Lynch MA, Dillon WP: Lesions of the head and neck in patients with AIDS: CT and MR findings. AJR 151:785–790, 1988.
5. Orofacial manifestations of HIV infection. Lancet 1(8592):976–977, 1988.
6. Drew WL, Mintz L, Miner RC, Sands M, Ketterer B: Prevalence of cytomegalovirus-infection in homosexual men. J Infect Dis 143(2):188–192, 1981.
7. Drew WL, Mintz L: What is the role of cytomegalovirus in AIDS? Ann NY Acad Sci 437:320–324, 1984.
8. Quinnan GV, Masur H, Rook AH, Armstrong G, Frederick WR, Epstein J, Manischewitz JF, Macher AM, Jackson L, et al: Herpesvirus infections in the acquired immune deficiency syndrome. JAMA 252(1):72–77, 1984.
9. Alsip GR, Ench Y, Sumaya CV, Boswell RN: Increased Epstein-Barr virus DNA in oropharyngeal secretions from patients with AIDS, AIDS-related complex, or asymptomatic human immunodeficiency virus infections. J of Infect Dis 157(5):1072–1076, 1988.
10. Greenspan D, Silverman S: Oral lesions: Dentists paly key role in early AIDS detection. CDA J 15(1):28–33, 1987.
11. Fung JC, Shanley J, Tilton RC. Comparison of the detection of herpes simplex virus in direct clinical specimens with herpes simplex virus—Specific DNA probes and monoclonal antibodies. J Clin Microbiol 22(5):748–753, 1985.
12. Gold JWM, Armstrong D: Infectious complications of the acquired immune deficiency syndrome. Ann NY Acad Sci 437:383–393, 1984.
13. Quinnan GV, Rook AH, Frederick WR, et al: Prevalence, clinical manifestations, and immunology of herpesvirus infections in the acquired immunodeficiency syndrome. Ann NY Acad Sci 437:200–206, 1984.
14. Seigal FP, Lopez C, Hammer GS, et al: Severe acquired immunodeficiency in male homosexuals, manifested by chronic perianal ulcerative herpes simplex lesions. N Eng J Med 305(24):1439–1444, 1981.
15. Cohen SG, Greenberg MS: Chronic oral herpes simplex virus infection in immunocompromised patients. Oral Surg Oral Med Oral Pathol 59(5):465–471, 1985.
16. Scully C, Cawson RA, Porter SR: Acquired immune deficiency syndrome: Review. BR Dent J 161(2):53–60, 1986.
17. Reichart PA, Gelderblom HR, Becker J, Kuntz A: AIDS and the oral cavity. The HIV-infection: Virology, etiology, origin, immunology, precautions and clinical observations in 110 patients. Int J Oral Maxillofac Surg 16(2):129–153, 1987.
18. Silverman S, Migliorati CA, Lozada-Nur F, Greenspan D, Conant MA: Oral findings in people with or at high risk for AIDS: A study of 375 homosexual males. J Am Dent Assoc 112(2):187–192, 1986.
19. Lozada F, Silverman S, Migliorati CA, Conant MA, Volberding PA: Oral manifestations of tumor and opportunistic infections in the acquired immunodeficiency syndrome (AIDS): Finding in 53 homosexual men with Kaposi's sarcoma. Oral Surg Oral Med Oral Pathol 56(5):491–494, 1983.
20. Green TL, Beckstead JH, Lozada-Nur F, Silverman S, Hansen LS: Histopathologic spectrum of oral Kaposi's sarcoma. Oral Surg Oral Med Oral Pathol 58(3):306–314, 1984.
21. Finkbeiner WE, Egbert BM, Groundwater JR, Sagebiel RW: Kaposi's sarcoma in young homosexual men. Arch Pathol Lab Med 106(6):261–264, 1982.
22. Lane HC, Masur H, Gelmann EP, Longo DL, Steis RG, Chused T, Whalen G, Edgar LC,

Fauci AS: Correlation between immunologic function and clinical subpopulatios of patients with the acquired immune deficiency syndrome. Am J Med 78(3):417–422, 1985.

23. Klein RS, Harris CA, Small CB, Moll B, Lesser M, Friedland GH: Oral candidiasis in high-risk patients as the initial manifestation of the acquired immunodeficiency syndrome. N Engl J Med 311(6):354–358, 1984.

24. Sooy CD: The impact of AIDS on otolaryngology—Head and neck surgery. Adv Otolaryngol Head Neck Surg 1:1–28, 1987.

25. Schofferman J: Pain: Diagnosis and management in the palliative care of AIDS. J Palliative Care 4(4):46–49, 1988.

26. Gabuza DH, Hirsch MS: Neurologic manifestations of infection with human immunodeficiency virus. Clinical features and pathogenesis. Ann Intern Med 107(3):383–391, 1987.

27. Wiselka MJ, Nickolson KG, Ward SC, Flower AJE: Acute infection with human immunodeficiency virus associated with facial nerve palsy and neuralgia. J Infect 15(2):189–190, 1987.

28. Langford-Kuntz A, Reichart P, Pohle HD: Impairment of cranio-facial nerves due to AIDS. Report of two cases. Int J of Oral Maxillofac Surg 17(4):227–229, 1988.

29. Astrom KE, Mancall EL, Richardson EP Jr: 1958, Progressive multifocal leucoencephalopathy: A hithero unrecognized complication of chronic lymphatic leukemia and Hodgkin's disease. Brain 81:93–111, 1958.

30. Gyorkey F, Melnick JL, Gyorkey P. Human immunodeficiency virus in brain biopsies of patients with AIDS and progressive encephalopathy. J Infect Dis 155(5):870–876, 1987.

31. Cornblath DR, McArthur JC: Predominantly sensory neuropathy in patients with AIDS and AIDS-related complex. Neurology 38(5):794–796, 1988.

32. Holmes VF, Fricchione GL: Hypomania in an AIDS patient receiving amitriptyline for neuropathic pain. Neurology 3(2 pt 1)305, 1989.

33. Shaha A, Thelmo W, Jaffe BM: Is parotid lymphadenopathy a new disease or part of AIDS? Am J Surg 156:297–300, 1988.

34. Smith FB, Rajdeo H, Panesar N, Bhuta K, Stahl R: Benign lymphoepithelial lesion of the parotid gland in intravenous drug users. Arch Pathol Lab Med 112(7)742–745, 1988.

35. Russotto SB. Asymptomatic parotid gland enlargement in diabetes mellitus. Oral Surg Oral Med Oral Pathol 52(6):594–598, 1981.

36. Hasler JF: Parotid enlargement: A presenting sign in anorexia nervosa. Oral Surg Oral Med Oral Pathol 53(6):567–573, 1982.

37. Holliday RA, Cohen WA, Schinella RA, Rothstein SG, Persky MS, Jacobs JM, Som PM: Benign lymphoepithelial parotid cysts and hyperplastic cervical adenopathy in AIDS-risk patients: A new CT appearance. Radiology 168(2):439–441, 1988.

38. Shugar JM, Som PM, Jacobson AL, Ryan JR, Bernard PJ, Dickman SH: Multicentric parotid cysts and cervical adenopathy in AIDS patients. A newly recognized entity: CT and MR manifestations. Laryngoscope 98(7):772–775, 1988.

39. Colebunders R, Francis H, Mann JM, Bila KM, Kandi K, Lebughe I, Gigase P, Van Marck E, Macher AM, Quinn TC: Parotid swelling during human immunodeficiency virus infection. Arch Otolaryngol Head Neck Surg 114(3):330–332, 1988.

40. Greenspan JS, Gadol N, Olson JA, et al: Lymphocyte function in recurrent aphthous ulceration. J Oral Pathol 14(8):592–602, 1985.

41. Antoon JW, Miller RL: Aphthous ulcers—a review of the literature on etiology, pathogenesis, diagnosis and treatment. J Am Dent Assoc 101(5):803–808, 1980.

42. Bach MC, Valenti AJ, Howell DA, Smith TJ: Odynophagia from aphthous ulcers of the pharynx and esophagus in the acquired immunodeficiency syndrome (AIDS). Ann Intern Med 109(4):338–339, 1988.

43. Silverman S, Luangjarmekorn L, Greenspan D: Occurrence of oral candida in irradicated head and neck cancer patients. J Oral Med 39(4):194–196, 1984.

44. Glick M, Cohen SG, Cheney RT, Crooks GW, Greenberg MS: Oral manifestations of disseminated cryptococcus neoformans in a patient with acquired immunodeficiency syndrome. Oral Surg Oral Med Oral Pathol 64(4):454–459, 1987.

45. Epstein JB, Truelove EL, Izutzu KT: Oral candidiasis: Pathogenesis and host defense. Rev Infect Dis 6(1):96–106, 1984.

46. Greenspan D, Greenspan J, Pinborg J, Schiodt M: AIDS and the Dental Team. Copenhagen:

Munksgaard, pp1–96, 1986.

47. Gottlieb MS, Schroff R, Schanker HM, Weisman JD, et al: Pneumocystis carinii pneumonia and mucosal candidiasis in previously healthy homosexual men: Evidence of a new acquired cellular immunodeficiency. N Engl J Med 305(24):1425–1431, 1981.

48. Tavitian A, Raufman JP, Rosenthal LE: Oral candidiasis as a marker for esophageal candidiasis in the acquired immunodeficiency syndrome. Ann Intern Med 104(1):54–55, 1986.

49. Greenspan D, Greenspan JS, Hearst NG, Pan LZ, Conant MA, Abrams DI, Hollander H, Levy JA: Relation of oral hairy leukoplakia to infection with the human immunodeficiency virus and the risk of developing AIDS. J Infect Dis 155(3):475–481, 1987.

50. Winkler JR, Murray PA: Periodontal disease. A potential intraoral expression of AIDS may be rapidly progressive periodontitis. CDA J 15(1):20–24, 1987.

51. Syrjanen S, Valle SL, Antonen J, Suni J, Saxinger C, Krohn K, Ranki A: Oral candidal infection as a sign of HIV infection in homosexual men. Oral Surg Oral Med Oral Pathol 65(1):36–40, 1988.

52. Murrah VA, Scholtes GA: Antibody testing and counseling of dental patients at risk for human immunodeficiency virus (HIV) infection and associated clinical findings. Oral Surg Oral Med Oral Pathol 66(4):432–439, 1988.

53. Greenspan D, Hollander H, Friedman Kein A, Frees KK, Greenspan JS. Oral hairy leukoplakia in two women, a haemophiliac and a transfusion recipient. Lancet 2(8513):978–979, 1986.

54. Greenspan D, Greenspan JS, Conant M, Petersen V, Silverman S, De Souza Y: Oral hairy leucoplakia in male homosexuals: Evidence of association with both papillomavirus and a herpes-group virus. Lancet 2(8407):831–834, 1984.

55. Conant MA: Hairy Leukoplakia. A new disease of the oral mucosa. Arch of Dermatol 123(5):585–587, 1987.

56. The American Academy of Periodontology: Current procedural terminology for periodontics, 5th ed., 1986. Rev November 1987:1–3.

57. The American Academy of Periodontology. Peridontal Therapy: A Summary Status Report 1987–1988. pp1–7, 1987.

58. Johnson BD, Engel D: Acute necrotizing ulcerative gingivitis. A review of diagnosis, etiology and treatment. J Periodontol 57(3):141–150, 1986.

59. Loesche WJ, Syed SA, laughon BE, Stoll J: The bacteriology of acute necrotizing ulcerative gingivitis. J Periodontol 53(4):223–230, 1982.

60. Sabiston CB: A review and proposal for the etiology of acute necrotizing gingivitis. J Clin Periodontal 13(8):727–734, 1986.

61. Dennison DK, Smith B, Newland JR: Immune responsiveness and ANUG. J Dent Res 64 special issue/abstact. 204:197, 1985.

62. Hydrogen peroxide—Use of abuse? The American Academy of Periodontology, October, pp 1–2.

63. Chemical agents for the control of plaque. The American Academy of Periodontology, April, pp 1–5.

64. Desai SD, Rajrathnam K: Laryngeal granuloma—An unusual presentation of AIDS. J Laryngol Otol 102(4):372–373, 1988.

6. CHRONIC PAIN SYNDROMES IN AIDS PATIENTS

RICHARD L. RAUCK

Since the physician's duty is to minimize human suffering due to medical and psychological illness, maximizing pain relief in HIV-infected people is paramount, especially given the fatal prognosis that AIDS carries. A person who does not describe classical pain is not necessarily free of discomfort, however. Paresthesias, dysesthesias, and burning produce significant discomfort and can be agonizing. These symptoms are difficult to treat since they do not readily respond to analgesics. Anesthesiologists use local anesthetic blocks to treat this type of pain in various illnesses, including reflex sympathetic dystrophy, herpes zoster and postherpetic neuralgia, peripheral neuropathies, and chronic pain of cancer. People with HIV infection may have significant pain with a number of illnesses. Management of those nervous system diseases with pain and dysesthesias, such as Guillain-Barré syndrome, predominantly sensory neuropathy, and herpes zoster, may be improved with regional local anesthetic injections. This chapter reviews these three chronic pain syndromes and their management, with special emphasis on herpes zoster.

GUILLIAN-BARRÉ SYNDROME
In a large public health hospital experience, the striking association of Guillain-Barré syndrome and HIV was demonstrated by the fact that 50% of those presenting with Guillain-Barré syndrome had concomitant HIV infection.[1] This is not surprising since it has been proposed that patients with immune dysfunction due to Hodgkin's disease or immunosuppressive therapy are at increased risk for Guillain-Barré syndrome.[2,3]

Guillain-Barré syndrome presents in people with HIV infection, as it does classically, with weakness as the major symptom and minor sensory loss.[4,5] Nerve biopsies reveal epineural inflammatory cell infiltrates with evidence of primary demyelination and axonal degeneration.[4] Some have shown phagocyte-mediated myelin stripping.[5]

Because AIDS is characterized by severe immunodeficiency, it may seem paradoxical that an immune-mediated neuropathy can occur.[6] This inconsistency may be explained as immunosuppression "triggering" an autoimmune disease.[3] Early B-cell activation after HIV infection results in increased levels of serum IgG and circulating immune complexes.[7,8] During this period the HIV-infected individual seroconverts.[9] Some have suggested that, along with other disorders, chronic immune thrombocytopenia and Guillain-Barré syndrome are immune-complex diseases.[10,11] In fact, both disorders clinically develop in the course of HIV infection. Further, antimyelin antibodies have been reported in an HIV-positive patient with Guillain-Barré syndrome.[12]

Most studied patients improved to normal over six months without treatment or with corticosteroids. After treatment successes with plasmapheresis, Cornblath and colleagues recommend it as the treatment of choice since corticosteroids may further impair cell-mediated immunity, contributing to other infections.[5]

PREDOMINANTLY SENSORY NEUROPATHY

Predominantly sensory neuropathy is a symmetric, distal, sensorimotor neuropathy found in up to 30% of patients with AIDS.[13] Painful soles is the most common complaint.[14] Usually a "pins and needles" sensation is described, although patients relate other "peculiar" sensations such as "a sense of cold water being splashed on my legs" or "a feeling of burning."[16] These "painful paresthesias" appear to be the most incapacitating symptom.[15] In contrast to Guillain-Barré syndrome, sensory symptoms predominate with little weakness.

The pathologic process is a progressive axonal degeneration or "dying-back" neuropathy. Recently, the finding of HIV-like particles in peripheral nerve axoplasm supports the etiology of a direct viral insult. Initially, there is a loss of axon related to defective axonal transport, followed by secondary demyelination due to immune abnormalities.[15] Dorsal root ganglionitis has been suggested to explain the dysesthesias.[5] Predominantly sensory neuropathy occurs without the characteristic remissions of Guillain-Barré syndrome.[15]

HERPES ZOSTER

The clinical significance of the varicella-zoster virus continues to expand despite the isolation of the virus over thirty years ago.[16] The host-parasite relationship has changed in varicella-zoster infections, and much of this can be attributed to medical progress of the past three decades. No longer can varicella-zoster be considered benign, especially in patients who are immuno-compromised or receiving cytotoxic agents. More recently, individuals with the acquired immune deficiency syndrome (AIDS) have been identified as high-risk patients for developing varicella-zoster infections. In these groups of patients, initial contact with the virus (varicella) or reactivation of the latent virus (zoster) can result in serious morbidity or mortality.

Epidemiology

While varicella infections remain underreported, contact with the virus extends to most individuals. In urban areas of the United States, the incidence of seroreactive individuals approaches 100%.[17] Estimates of 2.8 million cases per year exist, with over 80% occurring in children under nine years of age.[18]

For unknown reasons pneumonia and encephalitis, major complications of varicella, occur more frequently in very young children and adults. Over a recent five-year period, individuals over 20 years represented 1.8% of registered varicella cases but 24% of reported deaths.[19,20] While immuno-compromised patients account for many of the 100–200 annual varicella-related deaths in the United States, the incidence of complications in this group is not well documented.[18,21] Plebud did review the period from 1972 to 1978 and found 403 cases of encephalitis associated with varicella and 64 deaths.[18]

Epidemiologic data on primary varicella infections in AIDS patients are fragmentary. One would expect the incidence in young children, not previously exposed to the virus, to be extremely high. Fortunately, however, this group has remained too small to develop a clear trend. Most AIDS patients, and those at risk to develop AIDS, will have had a previous varicella infection, a result primarily of their age at diagnosis. One would also expect any primary varicella infection in these young adults to occur prior to the development and diagnosis of AIDS. At the time of its occurrence, a primary varicella infection in this population might not raise the same clinical suspicion as a subsequent zoster infection. This combination of small numbers and inadvertent underreporting results in inaccurate data.

Herpes zoster infections (shingles) represent a recrudescence of the latent virus. Frequency of zoster has been reported by Hope-Simpson at an attack rate of 3.9 per 1,000 population per year.[22] Further calculations of this population projected that half of all people living to 85 years would have a single episode of zoster and 0.1% would have two episodes. A different study yielded an overall age-adjusted incidence of 130 episodes per 100,000 person-years. Using these data it has been estimated that more than 300,000 cases of zoster will occur annually in the United States.[23] Postherpetic neuralgia occurred in 9% as the major complication of zoster infections.[24]

The incidence of herpes zoster infections in AIDS patients is elevated when compared with age-matched healthy individuals. More importantly, herpes zoster has been proven to be a clinical predictor for individuals at risk of developing AIDS.[25–27] Melbye and colleagues studied 112 patients who developed herpes zoster infections. The incidence of AIDS in the patients grew at an alarming rate of 1% per month. The cumulative incidence of developing AIDS after herpes zoster was found to be 22.8% in two years, 45.5% within four years, and an estimated 72.8% after six years.[27] They concluded that zoster can be regarded as an early indicator of impaired immunity and can serve as both a predictor of AIDS and a poor prognostic sign in patients at risk to develop AIDS.

On initial inspection, other studies appear to have different incidences; however, it is the long-term follow-up that tends to support the above statistics. Greenspan and colleagues showed only a 7% incidence of zoster patients developing AIDS, but their observation period extended only to 9–12 months.[28] A retrospective study of 300 AIDS patients revealed an 8% incidence of zoster prior to the diagnosis of AIDS.[26] The follow-up period for this group extended to 24 months.

In a Los Angeles study, 27 known HIV-positive patients with a history of herpes zoster were followed. Twenty-six (96% developed AIDS and AIDS-related complex (ARC) over a 3- to 42-month period, with a mean interval of 12 and 21 months for AIDS and ARC patients, respectively.[29]

Colebunders evaluated the effectiveness of herpes zoster as a clinical predictor in African patients. He listed a history of herpes zoster in 30 (11%) of 284 patients hospitalized for AIDS; 4 of this group reported a second episode of herpes zoster. He also performed serology on 146 patients with a history of a recent herpes zoster infection; 133 (91%) were HIV seropositive, of whom 23% experienced recurrences compared with none of the seronegative patients.[25] Unfortunately, no follow-up data were reported to evaluate the percentage of seropositive patients who would subsequently develop AIDS.

Herpes zoster, as shown above, can be used effectively as a clinical predictor for AIDS.[30] In 90% of the cases, the herpes zoster infection precedes the onset of AIDS. However, it has been difficult to predict accurately how early the herpes zoster occurs with respect to seropositive conversion. In Melbye's study the interval between seroconversion and herpes zoster ranged from 6 to 40 months (mean 23 months, median 32 months), but this actually underestimated the latency since all patients in this study were seropositive at the time of initial presentation. The only good data on this come from the Hershey cohort, where six hemophiliacs developed herpes zoster after enrollment, with a median interval between seroconversion and zoster of 58 months (range: 21 to 88 months).[27]

Pathogenesis

In the early 1980s Rogers and colleagues reported a cellular immunodeficiency in 52 patients with AIDS.[31] The patients were noted to have lymphopenia, increased levels of IgA, and reversal of the T-helper to T-suppressor ratio. Interestingly, the patients had significantly higher antibody titers to Epstein-

Barr virus and cytomegalovirus (CMV) but a lower prevalence of antibodies to varicella-zoster virus (VZV). Only 28 of 37 patients tested were found to have significant antibodies to VZV.[22]

These findings in AIDS patients produce a very favorable situation for reactivation of the varicella-zoster virus. A depression of cell-mediated immunity—in particular, a reversal of T-helper to T-suppressor cells—has been associated with herpes zoster infections.[32] Humoral responses have also been documented, with IgA and IgA antibodies detectable two to five days postrash and maximum titers achieved in the second and third weeks.[33] The exact mechanism by which the varicella-zoster virus exists quiescently after a primary infection has not been well elucidated. Evidence supports the hypothesis of the virus living in either one or more dorsal root ganglia. The virus–host relationship appears to be a dynamic process, the virus being kept in containment by humoral and cellular immunity and exogenous interactions with heterologous strains of virus. Rises in antibody titer have been reported in patients who have had a prior primary infection but not subsequent intermittent exposure.[34] Both normal and immunocompromised patients, however, maintain levels of antibodies indefinitely. This would not easily explain the recrudescence of the virus.[17] In contrast, cellular immunity begins to decrease after the fourth decade of life, leading to undetectable levels in some individuals. An inverse relationship has been noted between the incidence of zoster infection and the ability of the patient to mount an appropriate cellular immune response.

This decreased cellular immunity in "healthy" patients who have a recrudescence of the virus is also exactly what plagues the AIDS patient, patients with Hodgkin's disease, those with chronic lymphocytic leukemia, and immunosuppressed organ-transplant recipients. Therefore, a zoster infection in high-risk patients often signals the impending development of AIDS.[35]

Clinical course

Varicella-zoster virus produces two clinical syndromes: chicken pox (varicella) as the primary infection and shingles (zoster) as the recrudescent infection. Chicken pox most frequently occurs as a highly contagious primary viral infection in children. Initially, the virus infects the mucosa of the upper respiratory tract, predominantly the naces and oropharynx. An asymptomatic primary viremia results, with subsequent spread to the reticuloendothelial cells in replication. Following an inoculation period when the virus is disseminated by mononuclear phagocytes, a second viremia occurs, producing the prodromal symptoms and, finally, the cutaneous mucosal and visceral lesions characteristic of the disease.[36–39] Both humoral and cellular-mediated immune responses account for clearing the blood after the second viremia.

Complete extermination of the virus does not result during the primary infection; rather the varicella-zoster virus is able to travel from the skin and mucosal surfaces via neural routes to corresponding sensory ganglia. It subsequently lies dormant until reactivation takes place, commonly when a decline in immunocompetence occurs.[40] With reactivation the virus travels peripherally through the somatic nerves to the skin, resulting in dermatomal clusters of vesicles. Although pain precedes presentation of the vesicles, accurate diagnosis of a zoster infection usually awaits their appearance. See figure 6–1.

Most patients with AIDS will have already had the primary varicella infection. Thus the clinician will most always be treating zoster infections as the viral manifestation of this disease. A second primary infection of varicella can occur and has been reported, although not in the AIDS population.[41] Repeat zoster infections occur in all patient populations but have been more common in immune-incompetent patients, such as those with AIDS.

Complications

An uncomplicated course of zoster is characterized by vesicular eruptions and a moderate amount of pain along the affected dermatome. There can be complete resolution of the zoster infection without sequelae, more commonly seen in youner patients and immunocompetent patients. Immunocompromised patients, including AIDS patients, are considered at high risk for most complications of both varicclla and zoster infections.[42] Two studies of children with Hodgkin's lymphoma have reported the frequency of varicella infection at 22% and 35%.[43,44] A different series documented visceral involvement in 32% with a mortality rate of 7%.[45] Primary varicella infections have been noted to be uncharacteristically severe in HIV-infected children, with recurrence of an atypical, ulcerative herpes zoster infection.[46]

The frequency of zoster-related complications in AIDS patients differs from that of the normal population. In Melbye's studies severe painful zoster, involvement of the cranial dermatomes, and repeated episodes of zoster have all been associated with a poor outcome, hypothesized to be a result of the more severely impaired immune system.

While dermatomal zoster has been the most widely observed manifestation of the virus, dissemination can occur in the AIDS patient. How often dissemination occurs is not well known.[46,47] A disseminated state can progress from a dermatomal pattern, or it can occur in the absence of such lesions.[46] The disseminated state in AIDS patients can also be manifested as cutaneous, neurological, ophthalmic, and pulmonary.[35,36] Although gastrointestinal complications have been noted in the disseminated infection of other immunocompromised patients, visceral involvement has not been reported in AIDS patients.[46,48,49] Also, severe zoster infections in AIDS patients have been reported to result in more residual scarring than seen in other patients.[35]

In addition to increased severity of lesions, several case reports have documented an unusual form of disseminated ecthymatous varicella–zoster

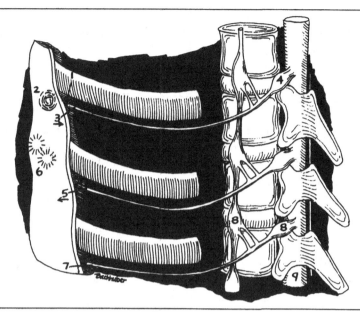

Figure 6–1. Varicella-zoster virus: Natural history. (1) Viremia. (2) Chicken pox. (3) Peripheral nerve migration. (4) Dorsal root sensory ganglion—latent station. (5) Reactivation; Peripheral nerve migration with resulting intense neural inflammation. (6) Herpes zoster vesicles. (7) Peripheral nerve migration. (8) With time, sensory and sympathetic ganglionitis. (9) Spinal cord and brain inflammation.

virus infection in AIDS patients. This form was characterized by necrotic cutaneous lesions during a prolonged course. The presentation did not resemble either primary varicella or disseminated herpes zoster infection; rather it was characterized by few vesicular lesions, central necrosis, and a tendency to persist and relapse.[50] These findings are similar to those reported by Gilson and Colleagues and underline the atypical presentation of common skin infections seen in AIDS patients. This atypical manifestation was associated with a severely impaired immune system in all four patients and inferred a poor prognosis.[50,51]

Neurological sequelae represent the most common complications associated with the varicella-zoster virus, particularly with herpes zoster infections. These can occur secondary to either local dermatomal distribution of the virus or through dissemination by the circulating system.

Postherpetic neuralgia (PHN) continues as the predominant neurological complication in immunocompetent patients with a zoster infection. PHN occurs during reactivation of the virus as it travels peripherally through the respective sensory nerves. The resulting nerve destruction can extend peripherally from a dorsal root ganglion (DRG), as a severe hemorrhagic regional ganglionitis in the DRG, or centrally into the spinal cord and brainstem. See figure 6–1. Peripheral nerve palsies, transverse myelitis, and ascending myelitis can complicate the reactivation of the virus within the dermatomal pattern.[52,53] Pain uniformly follows and is described as severe, burning, exquisitely dysesthetic and hyperpathic, and unremitting. Treatment, discussed later in the chapter, has been very difficult in patients who have had a neuralgia for more than one year.

The literature lacks data on the incidence of PHN in AIDS patients. It has been stated that the AIDS patient, despite a greater likelihood of developing severe painful or disseminated zoster, does not have a greater than usual risk of developing PHN. Since herpes zoster infections often occur years prior to diagnosis of AIDS, the development of PHN should be easily recognized. Nonetheless, only Friedman-Kien and Colleagues have reported a case of thoracic PHN in a series of 48 patients.[26] Melbye's group, and others studying patients longitudinally, have not specifically recorded the frequency of PHN.[27] No valid data have been published that compare the risk of PHN in age-matched zoster-infected AIDS patients with "healthy" zoster individuals. Other immunocompromised patients have been found to have a higher prevalence of PHN. We have felt that patients with AIDS, or at risk of developing AIDS, who develop herpes zoster infections should be treated aggressively to avoid both PHN and other complications of this potentially deadly virus.

While herpes zoster encephalitis can prove fatal, it often has a more favorable outcome when compared with other etiologies of encephalitis. Jemsik and colleagues' review of 39 patients with herpes zoster encephalitis provide a very good description of the clinical and pathological features of this complication, including mild confusion, hallucinations, delirium, headaches, and fever.[54] Rarely were there any focal neurological signs, seizures, or deep comas, although CSF and EEG abnormalities were often demonstrated. Neurological symptoms appeared as early as 7 days prior to, or 53 days after, the appearance of cutaneous lesions. The mean onset of CNS involvement was 9 days after herpes zoster outbreak, and the duration of neurological symptoms lasted approximately 16 days. Thirty-two of 39 patients survived the herpes zoster encephalitis, and most were reported to return to normal within one month. Unfortunately, 6 of the 7 who died were immunocompromised, a condition manifested in all AIDS patients. Further, 5 of the 6 patients were found to have disseminated disease.[54]

Herpes zoster encephalitis can manifest itself in several distinct patterns. The virus can produce a direct necrotizing encephalitis and myelitis, infecting primarily multifocal regions of white matter, and mimic progressive multifocal leukoencephalopathy (PML).[52,55–57] It can also produce a cerebral vasculitis that leads to thrombo-occlusive endarteropathy. Clinically, this condition occurs several weeks after eruption of ophthalmic herpes and is characterized by hemiplegia on the side opposite the herpetic outbreak. This vasculopathy involves branches of the circle of Willis and has been reported in at least one AIDS patient.[56,58] This condition quite possibly goes undiagnosed in some AIDS patients since it does not always follow a clinically apparent outbreak of ophthalmic zoster. It should be remembered that AIDS patients are quite susceptible to vascular insults, including thrombosis, infarcts, and hemorrhages; any cases of hemiplegia in AIDS patients should therefore list herpes zoster encephalitis as part of the differential diagnosis.[52]

Two cases of AIDS have been reported in which the encephalitis progressed as a chronic condition. One report revealed extensive ependymitis with periventricular extension and Cowdry A inclusions. In this patient the chronic progressive encephalitis extended for 18 months.[59] The other case involved a 37-year-old AIDS patient who developed central nervous system (CNS) disease 12 weeks after a course of cutaneous zoster infection and died two months later. In both cases the only organism cultured from the brain was the varicella-zoster virus. Interestingly, both patients (and a third without AIDS reported by Horton and colleagues) had developed two episodes of cutaneous zoster prior to the onset of CNS disease.[55] This may prove to be clinically useful in any patient who develops symptoms of encephalitis and has had two previous zoster infections.

In some cases of zoster infection, neurological involvement follows trigeminal infections of the first nerve division (ophthalmic). The herpes zoster ophthalmicus is often the only manifestation of the infection. As in other patients with zoster infection, this lesion has been suggested as an early marker of immune deficiency and later development of AIDS in patients at known risk.[60] A strong correlation has been reported in African patients between herpes zoster ophthalmicus and seropositivity in otherwise healthy adults.[61] Although no patients in these studies were followed longitudinally to see which would ultimately develop AIDS, reversal of T-helper to T-suppressor cells was found in five of seven patients studied and all five were found to have elevated immunoglobulin levels. The two patients with normal levels of immunoglobulin did not meet any AIDS-risk criteria.

Four other patients already diagnosed with AIDS had developed severe zoster ophthalmicus, characterized by prolonged cutaneous lesions, keratitis, and uveitis.[62] One final patient with AIDS developed vesicles of the eyebrow, nose, and lip and keratitis. The lack of any other ocular lesions led to a misdiagnosis of herpes simplex. Later, corneal scrapings cultured the herpes zoster virus and the proper diagnosis was made. Therapeutically, this differentiation is important since corticosteroids are helpful in zoster ophthalmicus but are contraindicated in herpes simplex lesions.[63]

TREATMENT

Guillain-Barré syndrome

Janisse and colleagues reported a case in which they placed an epidural catheter and continuously infused local anesthetic in a patient with GBS, but without HIV infection, who was ventilator dependent.[84] They were consulted because conventional treatment had failed to relieve his pain, which was largely from paresthesias and dysesthesias. They controlled these symptoms entirely with bupivacaine 0.0625% over ten days. This pain relief was considered dramatic by the patient, his family, the attendant nurses, and his internal medicine attendings. He discontinued the oral morphine, an anxiolytic, and a hypnosedative for sleep, yet he slept well and his mood elevated. Twice during his course when the infusion was inadvertently discontinued his previous dysesthesias returned, and in like fashion they remitted when the infusion was again begun.

In this case study the patient's previous morphine and sedative requirement was interfering with his ventilatory function. With thoracolumbar continuous infusion of dilute local anesthetic, the patient was much more awake, had more energy, and required less ventilatory support. They found no deterioration in his neurologic function; rather, his strength improved.

While this therapy is unconventional for patients with Guillain-Barré syndrome, this concept and approach of neural blockade by local anesthetic equal that for patients with herpes zoster and postherpetic neuralgia. Guillain-Barré syndrome may also be an ischemic process in part and may respond favorably to local anesthetic conduction blockade, which may also promote healing of the sensory ganglia, somatic roots, or peripheral nerves.

While Janisse et al. have not treated any AIDS patients with Guillain-Barré syndrome, its pain symptomatology is similar to that in patients with HIV infection. Epidural local anesthetic is a potential alternative therapy in an HIV-infected patient with Guillian-Barré syndrome or chronic relapsing inflammatory polyneuropathy who either is difficult to manage with conventional treatment or who presents with an unusual or prolonged course.

Predominantly sensory neuropathy

Only symptomatic treatment has been available for this painful, dysesthetic neuropathy, including tricyclic antidepressants, carbamazepine, phyenytoin, and topical capsaisin.[1,14] Schofferman, who manages people with advanced AIDS in a hospice setting, reported that of 100 consecutive people admitted, 53% had pain not directly treatable other than by analgesics.[64] In 36% the most common persistent or recurring pain was due to peripheral neuropathy. The symptoms described are those of predominantly sensory neuropathy, for which opioids alone are often unsatisfactory. Many people gain significant relief with a combination of an opioid and amitriptyline, in doses from 10 to 150 mg at bedtime.

We suggest that the application of local anesthetic block techniques, as discussed in this chapter, may be appropriate for some people with predominantly sensory neuropathy. If the neuropathic process can be modified soon after a diagnosis of predominantly sensory neuropathy, the resulting chronic pain may be reduced. Specifically, unilateral or bilateral lumbar sympathetic blocks or a lumbar epidural block would direct therapy to the lower limbs and quiet the pain and dysesthesias characteristic of this sympathetic-mediated pain. Any vasospastic component of the dorsal root ganglionitis and the immune-mediated demyelination could respond to local anesthetic neural blockade, in a similar way to the processes in Guillain-Barré syndrome.

Herpes zoster

Generations of medical students have been taught that no effective treatment existed for the varicella-zoster virus nor was it necessary as the infections caused by this virus were benign and self-limiting. This classical teaching has changed somewhat with Weller's review of the "not so benign virus,"[41] although many clinicians still do not offer treatment options to their patients unless a specific immunocompromised condition existed beforehand. While neither curative treatments nor any vaccines exist against the VZV, medications and anesthetic techniques have been employed to manage pain, shorten the duration of vesicular eruptions, and manage some of those complications described earlier.

Acyclovir significantly reduces the recurrence rate in AIDS patients with recurrent herpes simplex viruses; 44% of 300 patients taking 400 mg twice daily had no recurrences versus 4% in the control group. Although no statistics were reported in this study for AIDS patients with herpes zoster infections, a positive response was observed in patients given 800 mg of oral acyclovir five to six times per day. Topical acyclovir was also administered every two hours. Treatment was continued from five to ten days depending on the response. Patients reported decreased discomfort, diminished severity, shortened duration of lesions, and prevented or decreased scarring, which can be especially severe in the immunocompromised patient.[65]

Whether acyclovir can decrease the incidence of postherpetic neuralgia is doubtful. Separate studies by Peterslund and Bean showed no change in the incidence of PHN with acyclovir despite hastened skin healing and a shortened duration of both viral shedding and acute neuralgia.[66]

Pain management techniques

Treatment of herpes zoster in pain management centers and the utilization of anesthetic techniques have met with varying acceptance throughout the world. The Japanese have been extremely progressive and successful in managing early, acute herpes zoster infections.[18,67,68] In the United States management utilizing nerve block techniques has varied extensively. Educating primary care physicians on the merits of such techniques has resulted in appropriate referrals.

The pain of acute herpes zoster can often remain quite refractory to any standard medication regimens. Nonsteroidal anti-inflammatory drugs (NSAID) have produced good results, especially when inflammatory, hemorrhagic ganglionitis represents the major insult. They can also benefit any patient since the resulting neuritis from the zoster virus has an inflammatory component. Often, the highest recommended doses of any particular NSAID must be used because of disrupted blood flow to the vasa nervosum and compromised integrity of this vascular bed due to swelling and inflammation.

Tricyclic antidepressants (TCA), in particular, amitriptyline, have been used extensively in herpes zoster management.[16,41,69] While the mechanism of pain-producing stimuli differs between acute herpes zoster and PHN, the effectiveness of the tricyclic antidepressants depends on their ability to demonstrate rises in serotonin levels. This occurs by blocking the re-uptake of serotonin into presynaptic cells. A large interpatient variation in pharmacodynamics necessitates an initial low dose and titrating to effect. We begin with amitriptyline or doxepin at 25 mg at bedtime; for some patients, particularly the elderly, 10 mg at bedtime is sufficient. The long elimination half-life ($T_{1/2}$) of these drugs allows once-daily dosing, and the sedative qualities make bedtime dosing preferable. A single dose should not exceed 150 mg, although daily doses can escalate to 300 mg. We administer daytime dosing only when nighttime dosing has been maximized at 150 mg and the patient has no side effects or any change in analgesia. Daytime administration is maintained only if excessive sedation or other side effects are not produced.

Sedation has been the predominant side effect of tricyclic antidepressants but is beneficial when given at bedtime. Dry mouth can be an intolerable side effect in some patients but often is successfully ameliorated with lozenges. In some patients weight gain can be a significant problem and precludes their use. This issue is not seen in AIDS patients, whose appetite and nutritional status are often diminished. Tachycardia or other arrhythmias can be observed but usually are not clinically significant, particularly in younger patients.

For patients who cannot tolerate the tricyclic antidepressants, two other agents have been developed that resemble tricyclic antidepressants in their effect on serotonin levels but whose structures are different. Trazadone, a tetracyclic compound, has been very effective for use in AIDS patients with acute herpes zoster and PHN. We initially give 50 mg at bedtime but increase as indicated to 150 mg, with 1/3 taken at supper and 2/3 at bedtime. This drug appears to have analgesic characteristics similar to those of amitriptyline but is better tolerated.

Fluoxetine represents the most recently developed serotonin re-uptake inhibitor. Structurally, it does not resemble the tricyclic antidepressants but is classified as a phenylpropylamide. Lacking the sedative qualities of other drugs in this class, fluoxetine can increase many patients' energy levels. Dosing should be 20 mg once in the morning; if unexpected sedation occurs, then bedtime dosing can be recommended. Early trials for other patient populations have not shown increased effect with increased dosing; we have seen improved response in nonresponding AIDS patients when doses have been increased to 80 mg/day. We have also seen beneficial results when combining amitriptyline or trazadone at bedtime with fluoxetine in the morning. This regimen can avoid the "hangover" effect of the nighttime administration of tricyclic antidepressants and will elevate serotonin levels. It is cautioned that the combined use of these drugs can rapidly elevate serotonin levels fourfold in some patients and therefore must be monitored closely.[67]

Finally, we administer a tricyclic antidepressant or other serotonin uptake inhibitor for the analgesic effect, but we emphasize that they were developed for their antidepressant actions. This yields another advantage in a group of patients whose pain from the herpes virus, combined with an overall poor prognosis, commonly produces a clinically reactive depression.

Most patients with acute herpetic infections can be managed effectively with the use of nonnarcotic agents. Some will experience severe, often episodic, pain during the acute process that cannot be adequately treated without the use of narcotic agents. Patients who are immunocompromised and the elderly are more prone to severe outbreaks of herpes zoster infections and unremitting pain-related problems. The acute phase of herpes zoster infection is self-limited if complications are avoided, necessitating only short-term use of narcotics. The particular narcotic chosen depends on the individual patient status but often can be managed with a rather weak agonist such as propoxyphene or agents containing codeine and acetaminophen. In more severe cases hydrocodone or oxycodone will be efficacious. Since the refractory lancinating pain seen in severe cases is often described as episodic, "as needed" doses have been prescribed by the novice practitioner. This dosing regimen usually fails. "Around the clock" dosing with longer-lasting agents will be needed.

Those patients whose pain does not resolve during the acute phase will eventually develop postherpetic neuralgia. The mechanism of pain-producing stimuli of PHN differs from that of acute herpes zoster. Depending on the degree of neural damage caused by the virus, the locus for producing the pain will differ. Whenever extensive damage has occurred central to the dorsal root ganglion, the resulting pain can be expectedly severe. Severity worsens and becomes increasingly difficult to manage if the neural destruction extends cephalad through the spinal cord. Clinically, one cannot always distinguish the differing location within the neuraxis responsible for the virus-produced neuralgia although the efficacy of treatment will be significantly altered.

Medical treatment of PHN differs from that of acute herpetic zoster phase. Whereas the pain of acute herpes zoster usually lasts for a short, defined period, the pain of PHN can extend indefinitely. The pain in the acute phase is sometimes described with more severe descriptors than in the postherpetic neuralgia phase, yet the pain duration in PHN results in a much more debilitating illness. The intensity and duration of this pain produces in most patients the clinical signs and symptoms of reactive depression.

Tricyclic antidepressants have exhibited the best efficacy in PHN.[16,41,69] They elevate serotonin levels by blocking re-uptake, which occurs centrally and directly affects the descending inhibitory neural pathways coming from the brain and traveling into the spinal cord. Amitriptyline represents the prototypical drug in this class, and its analgesic efficacy is well documented. Unfortunately, its side effect profile precludes its use in some patients. It should be remembered that high antidepressant doses are rarely indicated, and if side effects are intolerable, the dose should be decreased prior to discontinuing the drug. We begin with 25 mg at bedtime but will decrease to 10 mg if side effects occur. If amitriptyline cannot be tolerated, a different TCA should be administered. Doxepin in equipotent doses has also been shown to have good analgesic potency in deafferented pain conditions. A tetracyclic compound, trazadone, and fluoxetine, a serotonin re-uptake blocker that differs structurally from antidepressants, have shown good effect. The potential benefits of tricyclic antidepressants necessitate trying several different agents before abandoning them. If a patient does not report analgesia on maximum doses of a single agent, we will combine any of the tricyclics with fluoxetine. As already described, this should be done cautiously as a fourfold rise in serotonin levels has been reported.

The NSAIDs have been utilized effectively in the acute herpes zoster infection but have not exhibited the same degree of benefit in the patients with PHN. A different pain mechanism is at work: In the acute infection the pain results from direct neural inflammation and active destruction of neural tissue. This type of pain can often be reduced with the NSAIDs. In postherpetic patients acute inflammatory changes are not ongoing, and so NSAIDs have less effect in this group.

Anticonvulsant drugs have not been frequently utilized during the acute zoster outbreak. Medications discussed earlier and anesthetic procedures have treated this stage effectively. The deafferent etiology of PHN results in neural overactivity, and this class of neural-membrane stabilizers is indicated in many situations.[16] Phenytoin has been successful in some and is prescribed in initial doses of 300 mg per day, which may be given at bedtime or divided into three doses. Although blood levels can be easily obtained, it should be remembered that they were designed for anticonvulsant conditions. If a patient has a therapeutic blood level but does not experience beneficial effects or side effects, the dose can be escalated to produce blood levels in excess of the maximum recommended values. Patients must be monitored more closely at higher doses for side effects.

Carbamazepine has been administered as an alternative to phenytoin. Some centers utilize it as a first-line drug for PHN. Like phenytoin, therapeutic levels often must be maximized or exceeded before effective analgesia can be obtained. Initial doses should be 300 mg per day in divided doses with escalation to 600–800 mg doses and occasionally beyond. The predominant side effects are sedation, nausea, vomiting, and dizziness. The rare but serious side effect remains aplastic anemia, which occurs in 0.1% of cases. Complete blood cell (CBC) counts need to be drawn at least every four to six months to monitor for this complication.

Capsaicin cream represents a promising new treatment for PHN. The active ingredient in hot peppers and related plants of the nightshade family, capsaicin is believed to react from blockade of terminal nociceptive sensory afferents from the skin. Small diameter nerves employ substance P, whose action is blocked with capsaicin. Several recent reports have shown capsaicin cream 0.025%, when applied to the skin four times a day, to be effective in the treatment of PHN.[68,70] A stronger concentration, 0.075%, is being used successfully elsewhere and is currently under development within the United States. The only side effect reported after the application of capsaicin is burning, occasionally so severe as to preclude its successful use.

Anesthetic Procedures

The preceding medication regimens have been useful adjuvants in the treatment of herpes zoster infections; however, they should almost always be employed in combination with appropriate regional anesthetic techniques. Only the most routine outbreaks of shingles in young, otherwise healthy individuals should be managed without anesthetic block procedures. All AIDS patients are immunocompromised and therefore at risk of developing delayed sequelae such as PHN, encephalitis, and dissemination. The acute herpetic attack is likely to be more severe and painful. For these reasons AIDS patients and patients at risk to develop AIDS should be treated aggressively whenever a herpetic zoster outbreak occurs. Treatment should be initiated at the earliest sign of infection to increase the chance of a favorable outcome. Since inadvertent puncture by a contaminated needle represents a known mechanism of acquiring the AIDS virus, all nerve blocks must be performed with extreme caution and respect for the increased risk encountered.

Several approaches to neural blockade have been advocated in the early acute stages of herpetic zoster infection. See figure 6–2. Regardless of technique, chances for a favorable outcome are enhanced if the neural blockade is performed early and repetitively in the disease process. High-risk patients, including the AIDS patient, require treatment as soon as lesions have been noted and possibly earlier whenever the presentation of pain can be described as classical symptomatology and the astute clinician feels comfortable making a presumptive diagnosis. Although injections prior to the outbreak of lesions have not been shown to benefit otherwise healthy patients, their early use in immunocompromised patients might prevent neural destruction and promote early resolution of the acute, painful zoster lesions.[71,72]

Blockade of peripheral nerve terminals has been reported to decrease pain and shorten the time to complete healing of acute herpes zoster vesicles.[73,74] Solutions of local anesthetics such as bupivacaine 0.25% to 0.50% in combination with a soluble corticosteroid, dexamethasone 4 mg per 10 ml, have been successful in our clinic. We inject beneath the lesions, using a 25-gauge needle; commercially available 2-inch and 3-1/2-inch spinal needles are available in 25-gauge sizes. For best results, injections must be kept

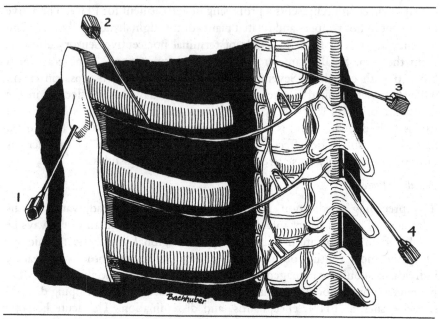

Figure 6–2. Site of local anesthetic blocks. (1) Subcutaneous infiltration. (2) Somatic nerve block. (3) Sympathetic ganglion block. (4) Epidural block.

subcutaneous in order to allow the injected solution to act at the nerve terminal. The corticosteroid reduces nerve inflammation in the surrounding tissue caused by the peripheral journey of the virus to the nerve ending. Bupivacaine anesthetizes the nerve ending and interrupts the pain cycle acutely and serves as a vehicle for the corticosteroid preparation. When infiltrating under the respective lesions, one should make every effort to deposit medicine under all involved areas. If pain is limited to one area of lesions, the remaining painless lesions should also be treated to prevent further inflammatory changes and potential painful neural destruction.

The frequency with which lesions need injecting has not been well elucidated. Some centers recommend daily injections, and others reinject every third or fourth day. We have had favorable results with injecting lesions every two to three days until all vesicles have sufficiently dried and no longer drain. When pain remains despite adequate scabbing of the lesions, we continue to inject for periods extending to two to three weeks. The need for prolonged injections does not often occur and should not be considered a failure of the technique. Perseverance in difficult cases can prevent delayed sequelae and complications, especially those seen in immunodeficient patients infected with the HIV virus.

Dissemination of the herpes zoster virus occurs more frequently in the AIDS patient, making it impossible to inject beneath all lesions. Nonetheless, some benefit and relief from pain can be obtained by injecting under selected painful lesions. Emphasis should be given to the most severe areas. Total milligram doses of local anesthetic can approach toxic levels in these situations. Manufacturers' recommended doses of corticosteroids should not be exceeded, in part to avoid further immunosuppression.

Visceral involvement of the herpes zoster virus has been recognized as an infrequent but bothersome occurrence. For obvious reasons, one would not be able to inject lesions involving nerves to the viscera.

Outbreaks of herpes zoster in the three divisions of the trigeminal nerve can produce severe pain and disfigurement secondary to scarring. While the pain of injection may be somewhat intensified in these locations, pain relief and enhanced resolution make injection desirable. None of our patients have been unwilling to have injections repeated when indicated. Corneal involvement, often seen in first division outbreaks, cannot be treated by this technique. Subcutaneous injections cannot reduce the inflammatory and destructive neural processes that occur proximal to the nerve endings. These destructive processes occur frequently since virus is sequestered in the dorsal root ganglion (DRG) during its dormancy.

The viral reactivation and eventual vesicular eruption occur after the virus has migrated from the dorsal root ganglion to the periphery. Resultant neural injury occurs along the respective pathway. Neural blockade along the somatic nerve path has been performed to shorten the healing time of vesicles and decrease pain. While any peripheral somatic nerve can be injected, the intercostal nerves are most often treated because of their frequent involvement in herpes zoster infections and the ease with which they can be injected. This technique has shown no advantage in adding corticosteroids to a local anesthetic solution. The local anesthetic will provide both analgesia to the affected dermatome and enhance circulation to the vasa nervosum. The vasa nervosum provides the blood supply to the nerve, and dilatation occurs through sympathetic blockade, seen with local anesthetic block of the respective somatic nerve. We perform peripheral nerve blocks with bupivacaine 0.5% and injection under the lesions. When combining these blocks, the peripheral nerve block should be performed before injection of the lesions. This allows analgesia of the involved dermatome and prevents any pain while performing subcutaneous injections of the vesicles. It should be noted that Raj has reported poor success with somatic nerve blocks. We would agree that somatic nerve blocks should be used only in conjunction with injections under the lesions. Long-term benefit from somatic nerve blockade may result primarily from the concomitant sympathetic block that occurs in most mixed nerves. Intraspinal nerve blocks represent an alternative to peripheral nerve blockade. Viral spread from the dorsal root ganglion can progress centrally into the spinal canal. Classical teaching reported that this phenomenon occurred later in the course of herpes zoster infection, but it may actually occur during the initial clinical manifestation. Whenever inflammation or neural destruction occurs proximal to the dorsal root ganglion, peripheral nerve blockade will not provide effective analgesia. Inadequate analgesia following a satisfactory peripheral nerve block can be considered diagnostic of central extension of the virus.

Epidural blocks are preferable to subarachnoid placement whenever an intraspinal block is indicated. Local anesthetics provide analgesia regardless of the route chosen, but subarachoid injection of corticosteroids is not recommended. Local anesthetics and corticosteroids are both indicated whenever an epidural is performed. A local anesthetic can provide almost immediate analgesia and enhance circulation to the vasa nervosum, while the corticosteroid will decrease any inflammation within the spinal canal. Only DepoMedrol® or Aristocort® should be injected; the water-soluble agents are contraindicated because of the highly toxic preservatives in these preparations. We commonly inject DepoMedrol® 80 mg with 0.125% to 0.25% bupivacaine (volume and concentration dependent on the locations of the lesions). Even though this depot corticosteroid lasts for several weeks once injected, most authors will reinject every two to four days with a total maximum of 200–300 mg of DepoMedrol®. Injections under the lesions should still be performed and preferably after the epidural block. Analgesia will then be established when the lesions are injected. Peripheral nerve blocks would be redundant if performed concomitantly with the epidural block. In patients requiring frequent blocks, however, we sometimes rotate the epidural approach with a peripheral nerve block.

Somatic nerves to the face can be blocked peripherally or more centrally at the trigeminal ganglion. This block is technically more difficult and can be avoided in many cases. Instead, a stellate ganglion block can provide analgesia and vasodilatation. Reports have shown that sympathetic blocks can reduce both the pain and vasospasm caused by the virus.[18,35,67,68] By promoting improved blood flow to the nerve, inflammatory and destructive changes will be decreased, toxic metabolites can be cleared, and resolution of vesicles and pain can be more readily achieved. These blocks can be repeated frequently in combination with local injections under the lesions. We currently employ high concentrations of local anesthetics (e.g., bupivacaine 0.5% to 0.75%), although others have reported success with a more dilute solution of local anesthetic.

The efficacy of sympathetic blocks for herpes zoster was first reported, in 1937, by Rosenak.[75] Twenty of 22 patients described had an extremely favorable outcome. Following this report, other studies showed not only excellent analgesia with sympathetic blocks but also a decrease in the incidence of PHN.[76] More recently, others have reported excellent results with sympathetic blocks during the acute phase.[77–82] Dan and colleagues reported that 210 of 213 patients obtained complete relief when they received sympathetic blocks within 14 days of skin eruptions.[82] While Dan found no cases of PHN, others have been no benefit of stellate ganglion blocks in decreasing the incidence of PHN.[79,83]

POSTHERPETIC NEURALGIA. Once the herpes zoster lesions have healed, pain should be resolved or decreased significantly. If pain remains, the patient must be considered at high risk for developing PHN; all AIDS patients with acute herpes zoster have an increased risk of developing PHN. The time from outbreak of lesions to development of PHN has not been clearly documented. The quality of pain often changes gradually, and most patients have difficulty remembering when the pain characteristics change. Within four to six weeks after an outbreak, the patient's pain begins to have characteristics of PHN, as described earlier in this chapter. At this stage the changes are still often reversible. An aggressive treatment, as already outlined, should be undertaken. At three months postrash lesions are well healed although further resolution of bad scarring will continue. The pain at three months, when present, is described as PHN. Nonetheless, nerve-blocking techniques have helped many patients when initiated at this latter date. When pain has persisted for one year prior to nerve blocks, all anesthetic treatment modalities have been discouraging.

We treat all patients with PHN of less than one year's duration with anesthetic nerve blocks. We prefer intraspinal nerve blocks, in particular epidural blocks, in this group of patients. We perform three epidural nerve blocks with bupivacaine 0.25% (6–10 ml) and DepoMedrol® 80 mg, injecting at the affected dermatome. These regimens can be repeated every two to three weeks. Corticosteroid can decrease any active inflammation within the spinal cord and aid in persistent hemorrhagic ganglionitis. If the initial block is ineffective, we rarely perform subsequent blocks in patients with long-standing PHN. Some patients' pain course can be very difficult to interpret after a single nerve block, and a second injection two to three weeks later may be indicated.

Rarely do sympathetic blocks benefit PHN since most neural destruction has taken place both centrally and peripherally. Epidural block with bupivacaine will block the sympathetic outflow at most given levels, with the exception of the trigeminal nerve and its three divisions. Stellate ganglion blocks have provided long-term relief in some of these unfortunate patients. In PHN patients who have become HIV positive, nerve blocks may decrease the likelihood of a second acute herpes zoster attack. While this has never been studied in AIDS patients, clearly, one would want to keep viable nerve tissue in its maximum state of health.

Somatic nerve blocks have been disappointing in this group of patients. Intercostal nerve blocks occasionally yield some early relief from pain, but they rarely give long-term relief. Further block of peripheral mixed nerves with a neurolytic solution should not be entertained. Although injection of neurolytics continues, most patients get very short relief, if any, and can often be left with a worsened dysesthesia after the block. Similarly, neurolytic intraspinal blocks have not produced consistently good results in these patients. When pain invariably returns and new pain complaints, commonly dysesthetic and hyperpathic, are often described by these patients, two to three weeks of analgesia cannot be justified in these patients.

SUMMARY

The varicella-zoster virus can no longer be managed as a benign entity. Patients infected with the human immunodeficiency virus and those with the acquired immunodeficiency syndrome have depressed immune systems and are known to be at high risk for developing potentially fatal sequelae from the virus. Their pain can also be severe. Increased incidences of dissemination and recurrent attacks mandate aggressive treatment. Specific therapies include intravenous antiviral agents in the hospitalized patient, possible long-term oral antiviral medications, oral and intravenous analgesics as indicated, and anesthetic nerve blocks performed early in the disease process and repeated as necessary to provide analgesia and prevent sequelae, particularly postherpetic neuralgia.

CONCLUDING COMMENTS

In the terminal phase of AIDS, people may experience great pain and suffering due to tumors, infections, or neuropathic processes. The patients may be seen on a hospital ward, in the ICU, in a hospice setting, or at home. We have had good results treating this terminal pain with methadone given orally or intravenously in a pharmacokinetic manner. Patient controlled analgesia and long term intraspinal analgesia have also been used with success in terminal stages.

Pain syndromes also develop in children although not enough data are available for review at this time. We look forward to covering this important topic in the future.

REFERENCES

1. Berger JR: The neurological complications of HIV infection. Acta Neur Scand 116(S):40–76, 1988.
2. Lisak RP, Mitchel M, Zweiman B, et al: Guillain-Barré syndrome and Hodgkin's disease: Three cases with immunological studies. Ann Neurol 1:72–78, 1977.
3. Drachman DA, Paterson, PY, Berlin BS, Roguska J: Immunosuppression and the Guillain-Barré syndrome. Arch Neurol 23:385–393, 1970.
4. Lange DJ, Britton CB, Younger DS, Hays AP: The neuromuscular manifestations of human immunodeficiency virus infections. Arch Neurol 45:1084–1088, 1988.
5. Cornblath DR, McArthur JC, Kennedy PG, et al: Inflammatory demyelinating peripheral neuropathies associated with human T-cell lymphotrophic virus type III infection. Ann Neurol 21:32–40, 1987.
6. Riggs JE, Rogers JS, Schochet SS, Gutmann L: AIDS-related neuropathy. West VA Med J 83:167–169, 1987.
7. Lane HC, Masur H, Edgar LC, et al: Abnormalities of B-cell activation and immunoregulation in patients with acquired immunodeficiency syndrome. N Engl J Med 309:453–458, 1983.
8. Gottlieb MS, Schroff R, Schanker HM, et al: Pneumocystitis carinii pneumonia and mucosal candidiasis in previously healthy homosexual men. N Engl J Med, 305:1425–1431, 1981.
9. Piette AM, Tusseau F, Vignon D, Chapman A: Acute neuropathy coincident with seroconversion for anti-LAV/HTLV- III. Lancet 1:852, 1986.

10. Clancy R, Trent R, Danis V, Davidson R: Autosensitization and immune complexes in chronic idiopathic thrombocytopenic purpura. Clin Exp Immunol 39:170–175, 1980.
11. Tachovsky TG, Lisak RP, Koprowski H, et al: Circulating immune complexes in multiple sclerosis and other neurological diseases. Lancet 2:997–999, 1976.
12. Mishra BB, Sommers W, Koski CK, Greenstein JI: Acquired inflammatory demyelinating polyneuropathy in the acquired immune deficiency syndrome. Ann Neurol 17:131–132, 1985.
13. Parry GJ: Peripheral neuropathies associated with human immunodeficiency virus infections. Ann Neurol 23(S):49–53, 1988.
14. Cornblath DR, McArthur JC: Predominantly sensory neuropathy in patients with AIDS and AIDS-related complex. Neurol 38:794–796, 1988.
15. Bailey PO, Baltch MD, Venkatesh R, et al: Sensory motor neuropathy associated with AIDS. NEUROL 38:886–891, 1988.
16. Weller TH: Serial propagation in vitro of agents producing inclusion bodies derived from varicella and herpes zoster. Proc Soc Exp Biol Med 83:340–346, 1953.
17. Gershon AA, Steinbert SP: Antibody responses to varicella-zoster virus and the role of antibody in host defense. Am J Med Sci 282:12–17, 1981.
18. Preblud SR: Age-specific risks of varicella complications. Pediatrics 68:14–17, 1981.
19. Annual Summary 1980: Reported morbidity & mortality in the United States. Morbid Mortal Weekly Rep 29(54):1–28, 1981.
20. Preblud SR, D'Angelo LJ: Chickenpox in the United States, 1972–1977. J Infect Dis 140:257–260, 1979.
21. Fleisher G, Henry W, McSorley M, Arbeter A, Plotkin S: Life-threatening complications of varicella. Am J Dis Child 135:896–899, 1981.
22. Hope-Simpson RE: The nature of herpes zoster: A long-term study and a new hypothesis. Proc Soc Med 58:9–20, 1965.
23. Ragozzino MW, Melton LJ III, Kurland LT, Chu CP, Perry HO: Risk of cancer after herpes zoster: A population-based study. N Engl J Med 307:393–397, 1981.
24. Horton B, Price RW, Jimenez D: Population-based study of herpes zoster and its sequelae. Medicine (Baltimore) 61:310–316, 1982.
25. Colebunders R, Mann JM, Francis H, Bila K, Izaley L, Ilwaya M, Kakonde N, Quinn TC, Curran JW, Plot P: Herpes zoster in African patients. A clinical predictor of human immunodeficiency virus infection. J Infect Dis 157(2):314–318, 1988.
26. Friedman-Kien AE, Lafleur FL, Gendler E, Hennessey NP, Montagna R, Halbert S, Rubinstein P, Krasinski K, Zang E, Poiesz B: Herpes zoster: A possible early clinical sign for development of acquired immunodeficiency syndrome in high-risk individuals. J Am Acad Dermatol 14(6):1023–1028, 1986.
27. Melbye M, Grossman RJ, Goedert JJ, Eyster ME, Biggar RJ: Risk of AIDS after herpes zoster. Lancet 1:728–730, 1987.
28. Greenspan D, Greenspan J, Goldman H: Oral viral lesion (hairy leukoplakia) associated with acquired immunodeficiency syndrome. MMWR 34:549–550, 1985.
29. Hardy D, Frankel LM, Gottlieb MS, et al: Varicella zoster virus infection (VZV): an early indicator of HTLV III induced immunosuppression. Second International Conference on AIDS, Paris, Poster 68, 1986.
30. Colebunders R, Mann JM, Francis H, et al. Herpes zoster and LAV-HTLV III infection in Africa, Zaire. 2nd Intern Conf on AIDS, Paris, Poster 328, 1986.
31. Rogers MF, Morens DM, Stewart JA, et al: National case-control study of Kaposis sarcoma and Pneumocystis carinii pneumonia in homosexual men. Pt Z. Laboratory results. Ann Intern Med 99:151–158, 1983.
32. Bertotto A, Bentili F, Vaccaro K: Immunoregulatory T cells in varicella. N Engl J Med 307:1271–1272, 1982.
33. Cradock-Watson JE, Ridehalgh MKS, Bourne MS: Specific immunoglobulin responses after varicella and herpes zoster. J Hyg (London) 82:319–336, 1979.
34. Brunell PA, Gershon AA, Uduman SA, Steinberg S: Varicella-zoster immunoglobulins during varicella, latency and zoster. J Infect Dis 132:49–54, 1975.
35. Wormser GP, Stahl RE, Bottone EJ: AIDS and Other Manifestations of HIV Infections. New Jersey: Noyes, 1987.
36. Arbeit RD, Zaia JA, Valerio MA, Levin MJ: Infection of human peripheral blood

mononuclear cells by varicella-zoster virus. Intervirology 18:56–65, 1982.
37. Feldman S, Epp E: Isolatin of varicella-zoster virus from blood. J Pediatr 88:265–267, 1975.
38. Gelb LD: Varicella-zoster virus. In: Fields BN, Knipe DM, Chanock RM, Melnick JL, Roizman B, Shope RE eds) Virology. New York: Raven Press, 591–627, 1985.
39. Gold E: Serologic and virus-isolation studies of patients with varicella or herpes-zoster infection. N Engl J Med 274:181–185, 1966.
40. Rosenblum ML, Levy RM, Bredesen DE: AIDS and the Neuro System. New York: Raven Press, 1988.
41. Weller TH: Varicella and herpes zoster. N Engl J Med 309(23):1362–1368, 1983.
42. Quinnan GV, Masur H, Rook AH, Armstrong G, Frederick WR, Epstein J, Manischewitz JF, Macher AM, Jackson L, Ames J, Smith HA, Parker M, Pearson GR, Parillo J, Mitchell C, Straus SE: Herpesvirus Infections in the acquired immune deficiency Syndrome. JAMA 252(1):72–77, 1984.
43. Feldman S, Hughes WT, Kim HY: Herpes zoster in children with cancer. Am J Dis Child 126:178–184, 1973.
44. Reboul F, Donaldson SS, Kaplan HS: Herpes zoster and varicella infections in children with Hodgkin's disease: An analysis of contributing factors. Cancer 41:95–99, 1978.
45. Feldman S, Hughes WT, Daniel CB: Varicella in children with cancer: Seventy-seven cases. Pediatrics 56:388–397, 1975.
46. Devita VT, Hellman S, Rosenberg SA: AIDS: Etiology, Diagnosis, Treatment and Prevention. Philadelphia: J.B. Lippincott, 1988.
47. Ebbesen, Biggar, Melbye: AIDS. Philadelphia: Sanders, 1984.
48. Figiel SJ, Figiel LS: Herpes zoster with ileus simulating intestinal obstruction. Am J Med 23:999–1002, 1957.
49. Wyburn-Mason R: Visceral lesions in herpes zoster. Br Med J 1:618–671, 1957.
50. Alessi E, Cusini M, Zerboni R, Cavicchini S, Uberti-Foppa C, Galli M, Moroni M: Unusual varicella zoster virus infection in patients with the acquired immunodeficiency syndrome. Arch Derm Atol 124:1011–1013, 1988.
51. Gilson I, Burnett JH, Jones PG, et al: Disseminated ecthymatous varicella zoster in AIDS. Presented at the Third International Conference on AIDS, Washington, DC, pp 1–5, 1987.
52. Harawi SJ, O'Hara CJ: Patholgy and Pathophysiology and AIDS and HIV-Related Diseases. St. Louis: C.V. Mosby, 1989.
53. Johnson RT: Viral Infections of the Nervous System. New York: Raven Press, 1982.
54. Jemsek J, Greenberg SB, Taber L, Harvey D, Gershon A, Couch RB: Herpes zoster-associated encephalitis: Clinicopathologic report of 12 cases and review of the literature. Medicine 61:81–97, 1983.
55. Horton B, Price RW, Jimenez D: Multifocal varicella-zoster virus leukoencephalitis temporally remote from herpes zoster. Ann Neurol 9:251, 1981.
56. Margello S, Block GA, Price RW, et al: Varicella-zoster virus leukoencephalitis and cerebal vasculopathy. Arch Pathol Lab Med 112;173, 1988.
57. Ryder JW, Croen K, Kleinschmidt-DeMasters BK, et al: Progressive encephalitis three months after resolution of cutaneous zoster in patient with AIDS. Ann Neurol 19(2):182, 1986.
58. Petito CK, Cho ES, Lemann W., et al: Neuropathology of AIDS: An autopsy review. J Neuropathol Exp Neurol 45:635–646, 1986.
59. Gilden DH, Murray RS, Wellish M, Kleinschmidt-DeMasters BK, Vafai A: Chronic progressive varicella-zoster virus encephalitis in an AIDS patient. Neurology 38:1150–1153, 1988.
60. Sandor E, Croxson TS, Millman A, Mildvan D: Herpes zoster ophthalmicus in patients at risk for AIDS. N Eng J Med 310(17):1118–1119, 1984.
61. Hornblass A, Jakobiec F, Reifler D, Mires J: Orbital lymphoid tumors located predominently within extraocular muscles. Ophthalmology 94:688, 1984.
62. Les Cole E, Meisler DM, Calabrese LH, Holland GN, Mondino BJ, Conant MA: Herpes zoster ophthalmicus and acquired immune deficiency syndrome. Arch Ophthalmol 102:1027–1029, 1984.
63. Engstrom RE, Holland GN: Chronic herpes zoster virus keratitis associated with the acquired immunodeficiency syndrome. Am J Ophthalmol 105(5):556–558, 1988.
64. Schofferman J: Pain: Diagnosis and management in the palliative care of AIDS. J Palliative

Care 4:46–49, 1988.

65. Conant MA: Prophylactic and suppressive treatment with acyclovir and the management of herpes in patients with acquired immunodeficiency syndrome. J Am Academy Derm 18(1):186–188, 1988.

66. Peterslund NA, Seyer-Hansen K, Ipsen J, Esmann V, Schonheyder H, Juhl H: Acyclovir in herpes zoster. Lancet 2:827–830, 1981.

67. Vaughn DA: Interaction of fluoxetine with tricyclic antidepressants. Am J Psychiatry 145:1478, 1988.

68. Watson CPN, Evans RJ, Watt VR: Clinical note: Postherpetic neuralgia and topical capsaicin. Pain 33:333–340, 1988.

69. Watson CP, Evans RJ, Reed K, Merskey H, Goldsmith L, Warsh J: Amitriptyline versus placebo in postherpetic neuralgia. Neurology 32:671–673, 1982.

70. Carpenter S, Lynn B: Abolition of axon reflex flare in human skin by capsaicin, J Physiol 310:69–70, 1981.

71. Yanigida H, Suwa K, Corssen G: Letters to the editor. Pain 34:315–317, 1988.

72. Yanigida H, Suwa K, Corseen G: No prophylactic effect of early sympathetic blockade on postherpetic neuralgia. Anes 66(1):73–76, 1987.

73. Epstein E: Treatment of herpes zoster and postzoster neuralgia by subcutaneous injection of triamcinolone. Int J Dermatol 10:65, 1981.

74. Epstein E: Triamcinolone—Procaine in the treatment of zoster and postzoster neuralgia. Calif Med 115:6, 1971.

75. Rosenak S: Procaine injection treatment of herpes zoster. Lancet 2:1056, 1938.

76. Milligan NS, Nash TP: Treatment of postherpetic neuralgia. A review of 77 consecutive cases. Pain 23:381–386, 1985.

77. Bonica J: Sympathetic Nerve Blocks for Pain Diagnosis and Therapy. New York: Winthrop Breton, 1984.

78. Colding A: The effect of regional sympathetic blocks in the treatment of herpes zoster. Acta Anaesth Scand 13:133–141, 1969.

79. Dan K, Higa K, Noda B: Nerve block for herpetic pain. Adv Pain Res Ther 9:831–838, 1985.

80. Gale DA: The management of neuralgias complicating herpes zoster. the Practitioner 210:794–798, 1973.

81. Higa K, Dan K, Manabe H, Noda B: Factors influencing the duration of treatment of acute herpetic pain with sympathetic nerve block: Importance of severity of herpes zoster assessed by the maximum antibody titers to varicella-zoster virus in otherwise healthy patients. Pain 32:147–157, 1988.

82. Dan K, Tanakak H. Kamihara Y: Herpetic pain and T-cell subpopulation. In: Bonica JJ, Liebeskind JC, Albe-Fessard D (eds) Advances in Pain Research and Therapy, Vol. 3 (Proceedings of the Second World Congress on Pain, Montreal, Canada. New York: Raven Press, 1979.

83. Tenicela R, Lovasik D, Eaglstein W: Treatment of herpes zoster with sympathetic blocks. Clinical J Pain 1(2):63–67, 1985.

84. Janisse T, Loar C, Raj PP: Pain in Guillain-Barré syndrome treated with continuous epidural local anesthetic. Unpublished data, 1990.

85. Bean B, Braun C, Balfour HH Jr: Acyclovir therapy for acute herpes zoster. Lancet 2:118–121, 1982.

INDEX

Accidental fall, 42
Acquired immunodeficiency syndrome, 1, 8, 9
  AIDS-related complex (ARC), 2, 8, 9
  analgesia (*see* Analgesia)
  clinical predictor, herpes zoster, 94
  diagnosis, 2–10
  education, 38
  etiology, 1–2
  long survivors, 29
  natural history, 55
  pathogenesis, 2–3
  pregnancy, 62
  prognostic sign, herpes zoster, 94
  psychoneuroimmunologic influences, 25
  women, 62
Acyclovir, 79, 101
Analgesia (*see* Opioids, and Anesthetic, local)
  AIDS, end-stage, for
  labor, 64, 67–68
  Cesarean section, 64
  PCA, 42
Anemia, 40, 45, 48
Anesthesia
  airway
    laryngeal lesions, 86
  caudal, 49

Cesarean section, for, 67
  Guillain-Barré syndrome, 46
cofactor, 38, 42
drugs, complications with
  enflurane, 41
  succinylcholine, 41
  muscle relaxant, 42
  nitrous oxide, 42
  nondepolarizing, 42
  opioids (*see* Opioids)
  oxygen, 41
epidural, 48
  abscess, 44, 45
  catheter complication, 46
  catheter technique, 51
  continuous, 48
  hematoma, 48
  epidural blood patch, 49
general, 37, 39–43, 47, 64, 66
immune system, 42
local (*see* Anesthetic, local)
machine, 54
management, 37
  agents, 38
  guidelines, 42
  plan, 39
  preanesthetic assessment, 38

obstetric, 63
  general, 64
    CNS depressants, 67
    immune response, 67
    muscle relaxants, 66, 67
    patient choice, 68
    ventilation perfusion, 67
  labor
    epidural morphine, 67
    Guillaiun-Barré syndrome, 46
    parenteral narcotics, 67
  regional, 65–68
  S.O.A.P. survey, 63
  local anesthetics, 64
  precautions, 68
  regional, 43–52
    coagulation abnormalities, 48–52
    complications, peridural, 44
    infection, 43–45
    parturient, for, 66–68
    neurologic disease, 45–47
  safety considerations, 52–54
  spinal, 48
    continuous, 48
Anesthetic, local
  bupivicaine, 46, 49, 100, 105, 107, 108, 109
  lidocaine, 46, 64, 75
  neurotoxicity, 45
  skeletal muscle, 45
  toxicity, 46
Anxiety, 4, 26
  (see also Depression)
Antibodies, 45
  antibrain, 17
  lupus anticoagulant, 49
  seroconversion, 92, 94
Arrhythmias
  azidothymidine, 40
  stress-related, 23
Asymptomatic, HIV, 2
Ataxia, 4, 47
Azidothymidine, 6, 53, 66, 77
  anemia, 40
  arrhythmias, 40
  mechanism, 6

Bereavement, 17, 21, 23
Behavior, 25
  biological links, 18
  immunology, 17
  interventions, 29, 69

limbic system, 18, 24
  stress, and, 21
  (see Treatment, psychological)
Biofeedback (see Behavior interventions)
Biology of hope, 28
Biopsychosocial, 16
  model, 30
Block, local anesthetic
  (see Neural blockade)
Bupivicaine, 100, 105, 107, 108, 109

Cancer, 23, 29, 49
  chemotherapy, 20
  multiple myeloma, 21
  oncologic viruses, 23
Candida, 2
  esophageal, 80
  oral, 75
Cardiac effects of HIV
  (see Nervous system, autonomic)
  arrhythmias, 23, 40
  cardiomyopathy, 41
  orthostatic hypotension, 41
  ventricular dysfunction, 40–41
CNS, clinical manifestations, 3
CNS syndromes, 4
  Aseptic meningitis, 4
  Vacuolar myelopathy, 4
  Progressive HIV encephalopathy of
    childhood, 4
  Chronic HIV encephalopathy, 4
  "AIDS dementia complex", 4
Clinical presentations of HIV, initial, 38–39
Coagulation
  activated clotting time, 48
  antibody, lupus anticoagulant, 49
  anticoagulants, oral, 49
  bleeding time, Ivy, 50–51
  coumadin, 51
  drugs that prolong, 50
  factor II deficiency, 49
  hematologic abnormalities, 49
  heparin, 48, 51
  partial thromboplastin time, 49
  peridural anesthetics, and, 48
  platlet count, 49
  prothrombin time, 49
  recommendations, for potential
    abnormalities, 50
  tests, 51
  thrombocytopenia, 48, 49, 92

thrombocytosis, reactive, 49
Cofactors, 26
  anesthesia, 38, 42
  behavioral, 27
  emotional, 27
  psychological, 26
  stress of surgery, 42
Consent, informed, 43, 47, 68
Corticosteroids, 99, 106
  dexamethasone, 105
  Depomedrol, 108, 109
  Aristocort, 108

Dementia, 4, 5
Depression
  altered immune function in, 7
  biological impact, 22, 28
  disorder, 24
  HIV encephalopathy, in, 4
  narcotics, and, 102
  presentation of HIV, 2
  psychological consequences of AIDS, 26
Diarrhea, 4, 9
Drug therapy
  orofacial
    analgesics, 78
    anti-bacterical, 84–85
    anti-fungal, 81, 84
    anti-viral, 75
  psychiatric
    lithium carbonate, 7
    monoamine oxidase inhibitors, 7

ELISA, 2
Emotion, 28, 31
  positive, 28–30
Encephalopathy, HIV, 2, 4–8
Encephalitis
  subacute, 2
  HIV, 4
Endocrine system (see Neuroendocrine)
Endorphins, 29
Epidural (see Anesthesia)
Ewing's provocative tests, 8

General anesthesia (see Anesthesia)
Gingivitis, 81, 82
Guillain-Barré syndrome, 8, 40, 91–92, 99–100

Hairy leukoplakia, 81, 82
Headache (see Symptoms)
Helplessness, 26, 28
Hematologic, abnormalities
  granulocytopenia, 45
  leukopenia, 42, 45
  lymphopenia, 1, 94
  thrombocytopenia, 48
Herpes zoster, 4, 8, 91–109
  clinical course, 95
  clinical predictor, 94
  complications, 96
  dissemination, 96, 106
  immunocompromised patient, 93, 95
  immunodeficiency, cellular, 94
  laboratory findings, 98
  neural blockade, for, 105–109
    caudal, 49
    epidural, 108
    intraspinal, 107
    intercostal, 109
    neurolytic, 109
    peripheral, 107
    somatic, 107, 109
    stellate ganglion, 108
    sympathetic, 108, 109
  neurologic sequelae, of, 97–101
    dysesthesia, 98, 100
    encephalitis, 98, 99
    ganglionitis, 92, 97, 101
    hemiplegia, 99
    peripheral nerve palsies, 97
    myelitis, 97, 98
    trigeminal neuralgia, 99, 107
  orofacial, 74
  pathogenesis, 94
  post herpetic neuralgia, 8, 97, 109
  prognostic sign, 94
  reactivation, 96
  treatment of
    anti-viral, 101
    anti-convulsants, 104
    bupivicaine, 100–109
    capsaicin, 105
    carbamazepine, 105
    corticosteroids, 99, 105, 106, 108, 109
    nonsteroidal antiinflammatory drug, 101, 104
    tricyclic antidepressants, 100, 102, 103, 104
    tetracyclic antidepressants, 102
  vasculopathy, 98

varicella-zoster, 77
viremia, 95
Holistic orientation, 26
Hope, biology of, 28–30
Hopelessness, 22–25, 28
Human immunodeficiency virus, 1
HIV–1, 1
HIV–2, 1
HIV
  acute, 2
  antibody seroconversion, 3, 9, 92, 94
  antigenemia, 3
  asymptomatic, 2
  children born with, 63
  clinical presentations, initial, 38–39
  encephalopathy, 2, 4–8
  latent, 38
  nephropathy, 2
  symptoms of (see Symptoms)
  tat gene, 26
Hypertension, intracranial, 41, 46, 47
Hypothalamus, 17, 18, 24

Idiopathic thrombocytopenia purpura, 2
Imagery (see Behavior interventions)
Immunity
  behavioral, 17
  cell-mediated, 2, 20, 74
Immune
  complexes, circulating, 9
  compromised patient, 74, 75, 80–82, 93, 95
  conditioning response, 24
  deficiency, 2
  modulators, 3, 17
  regulation, 9, 19
  thrombocytopenia, 48–50, 92
  transmitter, 25
Immunocyte, 31
Infection
  CNS, 43
  epidural, 43
  HIV, 45
Interferon, 3
Interleukin, 3, 19
Intravenous drug abuse, 9, 78

Kaposi's sarcoma, 2, 74, 75, 76, 81

Laryngeal lesion, 86

Leukopenia, 42, 45
Local anesthetic (see Anesthetic, local)
Lymphadenopathy, 2, 4
Lymphocyte, 1, 7, 18, 23, 25, 92
  natural killer cell, 18, 20, 24, 30
  stress modification, 16
  T4/T8 ration, 2, 76, 83, 84, 86
Leukopenia, 42, 45
Lymphopenia, 1, 94

Medicolegal, 38, 41
Meningitis, 4
Mental status, altered, 41
Monitors
  arterial line, 41
  central line, 41
Mononeuritis, 5
Morphine (see Opioids)
Multidisciplinary approach, 73
Myopathy, acute, 4, 5
  inflammatory, 9
Myelopathies, 4–5, 40, 47

Narcotics (see Opioids)
Nervous system, 2, 19, 65
  autonomic, 8–9, 19, 25
  central, 3
  pathogenesis of dysfunction, 2
  peripheral, 8
  sympathetic, 7, 17, 23, 29
Neural blockade
  caudal, 49
  Cesarean section, for, 67
  epidural, 108
  Guillain-Barré syndrome, 99–100
  herpes zoster, for, 105–109
  intraspinal, 107
  intercostal, 109
  labor, for, 64, 67
  local anesthetic, 8
  neurolytic, 109
  peripheral, 107
  Predominantly sensory neuropathy, 100–101
  somatic, 107, 109
  stellate ganglion, 108
  sympathetic, 108, 109
Neuroendocrine system, 19
  adrenal corticoids, 19, 23
  circuit, 7, 18

epinephrine, 18
pituitary-adrenal, 16
Neurohormones
  ACTH, 24
  CRF, 24
  FSH, 18
  GH, 18
Neuroimmunomodulation, 17
Neurologic
  complications, 2
  disease, 45
    demyelination, 6
    diagnosis, 6
    encephalitis, 44
    encephalopathy, HIV, 47
    meningitis, aseptic, 5, 44
    paraplegia, 45
    paresis, 47
    progressive, 45
    regional anesthesia, 45–47
    subcortical brain atrophy, 6
    vacuolar degeneration, 47
  initial presentations, 4
  peridural concerns, 46
  tests
    EEG, 5, 98
    CSF, 5, 98
    CT, 73, 78
    MRI, 6, 73, 78
Neuromuscular
  effects, of HIV
    paresis, 41, 47
    polymyositis, 42
  junction, 9, 41
  system, 9–10
Neuronal, dysfunction, 7
Neuropathy, 8
  autonomic, 4, 8
  chronic relapsing inflammatory
    polyneuropathy, 8
  diabetic, 9
  dying-back, 8, 92
  Guillain-Barré syndrome, 8, 40, 91–92,
    99–100
  immune-mediated, 8, 92
  inflammatory, 5
  inflammatory demyelinating
    polyneuropathy, 8
  ischemic, 8, 10
  multiple mononeuropathy, 8
  peripheral, 8, 77
  predominantly sensory, 8, 40, 92, 100–101

sensory, 5
sensorimotor, 77
vasculitic, 8
Neurotransmitter, 3, 10, 18
  dysfunction, 3
  peptides, 7, 24, 31

Opioids, 18
  endorphins, 24
  depression, 102
  morphine, epidural, 46, 49, 67
  methadone, 110
  opiates, 40
Orofacial
  endodontic infections, 85–86
  gingivitis, acute necrotizing ulcerative, 83
  hairy leukoplakia, 40, 81–82
  Kaposi's sarcoma, 75–76
  parotid enlargement, 78
  periodontal disease, 82–83
  stomatitis, recurrent aphthous, 78

Pain
  chronic syndromes, 91–110
  counseling, 69
  emotional factors, 68
  labor, 68
  neurologic (see Neuropathy)
  relief, postoperative, 38, 43
  terminal, 110
  transmission, 38
Pain Management
  Guillain-Barré syndrome, 46, 91–92,
    99–100
  herpes zoster, 91, 99, 101–108
  intraoperative, 39–52, 66–67
  labor, 67
  methadone, 110
  neurologic, 91
  orofacial, 73, 77, 79, 84–85
  postherpetic nerualgia, 109–110
  postoperative, 38, 43
  predominantly sensory neuropathy, 91, 92,
    100–101
  psychosocial, 28–29, 68
  terminal AIDS, for, 110
Paresis, 4, 41
Parotid enlargement, 78
Parturient (see Women)
Peridural

access, protocol for, 52
complications, 44
  anterior spinal artery occlusion, 43
  brainstem herniation, 47
  dural puncture, 47
  epidural hematoma, 44
  epidural abscess, 44, 45
  spinal nerve root injury, 44
  spinal cord injury, 44
  intraneural injection, 45
  intravascular injection, 44
  infectious contamination, 44
  dural puncture, 44
PMLeukoencephalopathy, 79, 98
Pneumocystis carini, 2
Post herpetic neuralgia
  (see Herpes zoster)
Predominantly sensory neuropathy
  (see Neuropathy)
Pregnancy
  (see Women)
Presentation, initial clinical
  (see Clinical presentations)
Procedures, invasive, 41, 53
Progressive multifocal leukoencephalopathy,
    77, 79, 98
Psychiatric, symptoms, 4
Psychoneuroimmunology (PNI)
  AIDS, and, 25–28
  circuit, 7
  conditioning of immune response, 20–21
  historical review, 16–17
  hope, biology of, 28–30
  hopelessness, 22–25
  hypothesis, 15
  neuroimmunomodulation, 17–21
  neurotransmitter dysfunction, 3
Psychological
  interventions, 30
  hardiness, 30
Psychosocial responses, 27
  support, 28
  factors, 30
  biopsychosocial, 30

Safety considerations, 52–55
Seizures, 4, 5, 41, 98
Seroconversion, 3, 9, 92, 94
Stress, 21
  concepts, 22
  control, 22, 26, 30

coping mechanisms, 21
death, 23, 24
hypersensitivity reaction, 18
immune system, and, 21–22
infectious mononucleosis, 17
lymphocyte change, 16
surgery, of, 49
sympathetic nervous system
  (see Nervous system, sympathetic)
vagal discharge, 23
Stomatitis aphthous, 78–79
Sympathetic nervous system
  (see Nervous system, sympathetic)
Symptoms, of HIV
  physical, 3–4, 41–47
  presenting, 3–4, 39–41
  psychobehavioral, 4
  psychiatric
    psychosis, acute, 4
    schizophrenia, 17
Sweats, night, 4, 9

T4/T8 ratio, 2, 76, 83, 84, 86
Transfusion, blood (see Transmission)
Transmission, HIV, 61
  anesthetic machine, 54
  blood
    aerosolized, 43
    transfusion, 52, 82
  breast feeding, 63
  hemophiliac, 82
  heterosexual, 61
  intravenous drug abuse, 61
  needles, 53
  peridural, 52
  perinatal, 62
  pregnant women, 54
  risk, 61
  saliva, 54
  sputum, 54
  transplacental, 63
Treatment, psychological
  counseling, 28
  psychotherapy, 28
  imagery, 29
  biofeedback, 29
Tricyclic antidepressants
  amitriptyline, 100, 102–104
  doxepin, 102, 104
Trophism
  lymphotrophic, 3

neurotrophic, 3, 42

Universal precautions 53–54

Vasa nervosum, 102, 107
Virus
  cytomegalovirus, 26, 95
  Epstein-Barr, 27, 74, 94
  herpes simplex, 26, 67, 74, 77
  herpes zoster
    (*see* Herpes zoster)

Western blot, 2
Women
  AIDS, and, 62
  education, 62
  pregnancy
    AIDS, and, 62–63
    anesthesia, and, 63–68
      (*also see* Anesthesia)
    cytomegalovirus, 54, 67
    herpes simplex, 67
    immunosuppressive, 63